Problem Solving in
Women's Health

MARGARET REES MA, DPhil, FRCOG
Reader in Reproductive Medicine, Honorary Consultant in Medical Gynaecology,
Women's Centre, John Radcliffe Hospital, Oxford, UK

SALLY HOPE FRCGP, DRCOG
Department of Primary Health Care, University of Oxford, Oxford, UK

MARTIN K OEHLER MD, PhD, FRANZCOG
Department of Gynaecological Oncology, Royal Adelaide Hospital, Adelaide, Australia

JANE MOORE MRCOG
Honorary Consultant Gynaecologist, Nuffield Department of Obstetrics and Gynaecology,
John Radcliffe Hospital, Oxford, UK

POLLY CRAWFORD MRCGP, DFFP
Women's Centre, John Radcliffe Hospital, Oxford, UK

CLINICAL PUBLISHING

OXFORD

CLINICAL PUBLISHING
an imprint of Atlas Medical Publishing Ltd
Oxford Centre for Innovation
Mill Street, Oxford OX2 0JX, UK

tel: +44 1865 811116
fax: +44 1865 251550

email: info@clinicalpublishing.co.uk
web: www.clinicalpublishing.co.uk

Distributed in USA and Canada by:
Clinical Publishing
30 Amberwood Parkway
Ashland OH 44805 USA
tel: 800-247-6553 (toll free within US and Canada)
fax: 419-281-6883
email: order@bookmasters.com

Distributed in UK and Rest of World by:
Marston Book Services Ltd
PO Box 269
Abingdon
Oxon OX14 4YN
UK
tel: +44 1235 465500
fax: +44 1235 465555
email: trade.orders@marston.co.uk

Although every effort has been made to ensure that all owners of
copyright material have been acknowledged in this publication, we
would be glad to acknowledge in subsequent reprints or editions any
omissions brought to our attention.

A catalogue record for this book is available from the British Library.

ISBN 13   978 1 84692 028 8
ISBN 10   1 84692 028 0

The publisher makes no representation, express or implied, that the
dosages in this book are correct. Readers must therefore always check
the product information and clinical procedures with the most up-to-
date published product information and data sheets provided by the
manufacturers and the most recent codes of conduct and safety
regulations. The authors and the publisher do not accept any liability
for any errors in the text or for the misuse or misapplication of
material in this work.

Project manager: Gavin Smith, GPS Publishing Solutions, Herts, UK
Typeset by Phoenix Photosetting, Chatham, UK
Printed by TG Hostench S. A., Barcelona

Contents

Abbreviations

Abbreviation:	Chapter(s):	Definition:
ACOG	9,46	American College of Obstetricians and Gynecologists
ACS	41	American Cancer Society
ACTs	10	alternative and complementary therapies
AFC	18	antral follicle count
AIS	7	androgen insensitivity syndrome
AMH	18	anti-Müllerian hormone
ART	19	assisted reproduction treatment
BMD	5,13,24,25,44	bone mineral density
BMI	8,20	body mass index
BTX	37,39	botulinum toxin
BV	32	bacterial vaginosis
CAI	38	community acquired infection
CBT	33	cognitive behavioural therapy
CCCT	18	Clomiphene Citrate Challenge Test
CFU	38	colony-forming units
CI	5,16,21,23	confidence interval
CIN	41,48	cervical intraepithelial neoplasia
COC	1,5,11,16,23,25,29, 32,43	combined oral contraceptive
COX	1	cyclooxygenase
COX-1	1	cyclooxygenase-1
COX-2	1,3	cyclooxygenase-2
CPP	4	Chronic pelvic pain
CT	45,47,48,49	computed tomography
D&C	14,46	dilatation and curettage
DES	14	diethylstilbestrol
DEXA	13,44	dual-energy X-ray absorptiometry
DHEA	17,30	dehydroepiandrosterone
DMPA	24,25	depot medroxyprogesterone acetate
DSM-IV	31	Diagnostic and Statistical Manual of Mental Disorders–Fourth Edition
DVS	15	desvenlafaxine succinate
EA	2	endometrial ablation
EFORT	18	exogenous FSH ovarian reserve test
ERMD	7	exercise related menstrual dysfunction
ERPC	26	evacuation of retained products of conception
EUA	45	examination under anaesthesia
FDA	1,14,43,46	Food and Drug Administration
FIGO	45,46,48,49	International Federation of Gynaecology and Obstetrics
FSH	7,11,12,18,19,22,25	follicle-stimulating hormone
GAST	18	gonadotrophin agonist stimulation test
GnRH	1,4,5,6,7,19	gonadotrophin-releasing hormone
GnRHa	5	gonadotrophin-releasing hormone agonist

Abbreviation:	Chapter(s):	Definition:
GTD	28	gestational trophoblastic disease
hCG	19,26,27	human chorionic gonadotrophin
HERS	16	Heart and Estrogen/progestin Replacement Study
HGSIL	45	high-grade squamous intraepithelial lesion
HIV	34,35,41	human immunodeficiency virus
HNPCC	50	hereditary non-polyposis colorectal cancer
HPV	41,45	human papillomavirus
HRT	2,11,12,13, 14,15, 16,17,40,42,46,50	hormone replacement therapy
HSG	18	hysterosalpingogram
HSV	35	herpes simplex virus
IBS	4	irritable bowel syndrome
IC	4,39	interstitial cystitis
ICSI	19,21	intracytoplasmic sperm injection
Ig	22	immunoglobulin
IP	49	intraperitoneal (chemotherapy)
ISVD	48	International Society for the Study of Vulvar Disease
IU	18	international units
IUCD	29	intrauterine contraceptive device
IUI	19	intrauterine insemination
IUS	1	intrauterine system
IVF	5,19,27	*in vitro* fertilization
LACE	46	Laparascopic Approach to Cancer of the Endometrium
LAP2	46	Laparascopic Surgery or Standard Surgery in Treating Patients with Endometrial Cancer or Cancer of the Uterus
LBC	41	liquid-based cytology
LH	7,18,22	luteinizing hormone
LNG	1,29	levonorgestrel
LNG-IUS	1,6,11,12,25	levonorgestrel-releasing intrauterine system
LUNA	3	laparoscopic uterine nerve ablation
LVSI	45,46	lymphovascular space invasion
MEA	2	microwave endometrial ablation
MPA	46	medroxyprogesterone acetate
MRI	3,4,7,22,42,45, 46,48	magnetic resonance imaging
MSU	37,38	mid-stream urine
NAAT	35	nucleic acid amplification technique
NCI	43	National Cancer Institute
NICE	42	National Institute for Clinical Excellence
NIH-NIDDK	39	National Institutes of Health – National Institute of Diabetes and Digestive and Kidney Diseases
NSAID	1,3,5,6,20	non-steroidal anti-inflammatory drug
OAB	37	overactive bladder
OR	16,21	odds ratio
ORT	18	ovarian reserve test
OVVOL	18	ovarian volume
PCO	7	polycystic ovaries
PCOS	8,20,46	polycystic ovary syndrome
PEPI	42	Progestin Estrogen–Progestin Intervention
PET	45	positron emission tomography
PFMT	36	pelvic floor muscle training

Abbreviation:	Chapter(s):	Definition:
PGF2	10	prostaglandin F2
PID	18,35	pelvic inflammatory disease
PMB	14	post-menopausal bleeding
PSN	3	presacral neurectomy
PMS	9	premenstrual syndrome
POC	25	progesterone-only contraception
POF	12	premature ovarian failure
PTH	13	parathyroid hormone
PUFAs	10	polyunsaturated fatty acids
PVA	6	polyvinyl alcohol
PYC	10	pycnogenol
RANKL	13	receptor activator of nuclear factor-kappa B ligand
RCT	13	randomized controlled trial
REA	2	rollerball endometrial ablation
SD	44	standard deviations
SERM	13	selective oestrogen receptor modulator
SNRI	15,36	serotonin and noradrenaline reuptake inhibitor
SPRM	6	selective progesterone receptor modulator
SSRIs	9,15,30	selective serotonin reuptake inhibitors
STIs	24,25,29,32,35,40	sexually transmitted infections
T3	28	triiodothyronine
T4	28	thyroxine
TAHBSO	46,50	total abdominal hysterectomy and bilateral salpingo-oophorectomy
TCRE	2	transcervical endometrial resection
TOP	4,23,29	termination of pregnancy
TSH	28	thyroid-stimulating hormone
TVS	11,14,22,23,26,27,43	transvaginal ultrasound scanning
TVT	36	tension-free vaginal tape
UAE	6	uterine artery embolization
UK	24,29,35,42,44	United Kingdom
UPSI	29	unprotected sexual intercourse
US	10,35	United States
UTI	38	urinary tract infection
VAC	10	vitex agnus castus
VEGF	47	vascular endothelial growth factor
VIN	48	vulvar intraepithelial neoplasia
VTE	16	venous thromboembolism
VVC	34	vulvovaginal candidiasis
WHI	13,16,42	Women's Health Initiative
WHO	18,24,25	World Health Organization
WHOMEC	25	World Health Organization Medical Eligibility Criteria for Contraceptive Use

Preface

Problem solving in women's health aims to give health professionals an easily readable practical guide to deal with common gynaecological presentations. The evidence, where available, is presented. With the lifespan of women continuing to increase and many surviving into their 10th or even 11th decades the problems of postreproductive health are increasing. This book covers problems from the menarche until old age.

The book is in eight sections and covers menstrual problems, menopause, fertility and contraception, gynaecological emergencies, sexual problems, urogenital problems, prevention and screening and gynaecological cancer. Alternative and complementary therapies as well as standard pharmacopiea are discussed.

The cases are described in a format suitable both for a consultation and could also be used for teaching and training of medical postgraduates preparing for higher qualifications. The cases are based on common problems encountered by the authors in both primary care and hospital-based practice.

Margaret Rees
Sally Hope
Jane Moore
Polly Crawford
Martin Oehler
October 2007

Acknowledgements

The authors would like to thank both Drs Ingrid Granne and Katy Vincent (Nuffield Department of Obstetrics and Gynaecology, Oxford) for their help.

Menstrual Problems

PROBLEM

01 Menorrhagia with Medical Management

Case History

A 35-year-old woman comes complaining that her periods have become increasingly heavy since her children were born. She stopped the pill, which in the past had made her periods lighter, and is now using condoms for contraception. She does not want surgery.

How do you assess her?

What are the non-hormonal treatment options?

What are the hormonal options?

Background

Menorrhagia is a complaint of heavy cyclical menstrual blood loss over several consecutive cycles without any intermenstrual or post-coital bleeding.[1] In objective terms it is a blood loss greater than 80 ml per period.[2] While various pathologies have been implicated in menorrhagia, in 50% of cases of objective menorrhagia no pathology is found at hysterectomy. Although 'unexplained' menorrhagia is a very appropriate term, the label dysfunctional uterine bleeding, which implies endocrine abnormalities, is often given. However most cases of menorrhagia are associated with regular ovulatory cycles, and anovular cycles tend mainly to occur soon after the menarche or in the peri-menopausal period. Management has changed over the past two decades with the introduction of the levonorgestrel-releasing intrauterine device. In the United Kingdom the number of hysterectomies for menorrhagia fell by 36% between 1989 and 2002/3.[3] Medical management is advocated as initial treatment in women without significant pelvic pathology.[2,4]

How do you assess her?

Patients with menorrhagia commonly complain of increased menstrual loss requiring more sanitary protection or the passage of clots and flooding. History and assessment are detailed in Table 1.1.

Table 1.1 History and assessment
What questions do you ask?
● Duration of the problem
● Flooding or passage of clots
● Length and frequency of periods
● Has there been any change
● Intermenstrual bleeding or post-coital bleeding
● Presence of pelvic pain or dyspareunia
● Contraception used
● Are cervical smears up to date (according to local screening programmes)
Assessment
● Undertake pelvic examination and cervical smear (according to local screening programmes)
● Haematology and biochemistry
● Imaging
● Endometrial sampling
● Hysteroscopy

In a woman of this age pelvic pathology is unlikely so if pelvic examination is normal and there are no other symptoms, one can proceed to treat her medically. It is essential to check that she is not anaemic but further tests such as thyroid function should only be undertaken if clinically indicated. However if she does not respond to treatment she will need further investigation starting with a transvaginal ultrasound scan.

What are the non-hormonal treatment options?

Non-steroidal anti-inflammatory drugs

The cyclooxygenase (COX) pathway, with its two enzymes cyclooxygenase-1 (COX-1) and cyclooxygenase-2 (COX-2), represents one of the major routes for oxidative metabolism of arachidonic acid to prostaglandins. Cyclooxygenase inhibitors, commonly referred to as non-steroidal anti-inflammatory drugs (NSAIDs), can be chemically classified into two main groups: COX-1 inhibitors (salicylates [aspirin], indoleacetic acid analogues [indomethacin], aryl propionic acid derivatives [naproxen, ibuprofen] and fenamates [mefenamic acid, flufenamic acid, meclofenamic acid]) and COX-2 inhibitors (coxibs [celecoxib]).

Various NSAIDs have been evaluated in a number of randomized trials, which have to date been limited to COX-1 inhibitors. In a Cochrane review, five of seven randomized trials showed that mean menstrual blood loss was less with NSAIDs than with placebo, and two showed no difference.[5] Furthermore, there was no evidence that one NSAID (naproxen or mefenamic acid) was superior to the other. The fenamates (e.g. mefenamic acid) are the most extensively studied NSAIDs. They have the unique property of inhibiting prostaglandin synthesis as well as binding to prostaglandin receptors, whose concentrations are significantly increased in the uteri of women with menorrhagia.[1] The percentage of blood loss reduction varies from 25% to 47% depending on the agent and dosage used.[5] An additional beneficial effect is that these drugs will also alleviate symptoms of dysmenorrhoea.

Optimal doses and schedules are difficult to define. Most studies, however, analyzed regimens starting on the first day of menstruation and continuing for five days or until cessation of menstruation. Common side effects of NSAIDs are gastrointestinal irritation and inhibition of platelet aggregation. Specific inhibitors of COX-2 might also be effective in the treatment of menorrhagia, but there is great uncertainty about the safety of this class of drugs.

Antifibrinolytics

Plasminogen activator inhibitors have been promoted as a treatment for menorrhagia because of increased endometrial fibrinolytic activity in women with menorrhagia. Tranexamic acid 2–4.5 g/day for four to seven days reduces menstrual blood flow by between 34% to 59% over two to three cycles. The effect is superior to placebo, mefenamic acid, flurbiprofen, ethamsylate and oral luteal phase norethisterone at clinically relevant dosages.[6] Side effects are mainly limited to mild gastrointestinal complaints. Earlier theoretical concerns about thromboembolism caused by the antifibrinolytic action of tranexamic acid have been refuted by long-term studies.

Etamsylate

Etamsylate is thought to act by reducing capillary fragility, though the precise mechanisms are uncertain. Studies with objective menstrual blood loss measurement using the currently recommended doses show that it is ineffective.[4]

Hormonal treatments

Progestogens

The use of progestogens is based on the erroneous concept that women with menorrhagia principally have anovulatory cycles and that a progestogen supplement is required. Progestogens are a common prescription for women complaining of menorrhagia. Oral administration, intrauterine administration and intramuscular depot injections are employed. The latter are used mainly for contraception and there is little information regarding menorrhagia.

Intrauterine administration

Intrauterine administration, especially of levonorgestrel (LNG), is very effective. There are currently two progestogen-impregnated devices: the Mirena® intrauterine system (IUS), which delivers 20 µg of LNG over 24 hours for about five years and the Progestasert® IUS, which releases about 65 µg of progesterone over 24 hours for about 16 months. Other newer, so-called 'frameless' IUSs are currently being evaluated.

The Mirena® levonorgestrel-releasing intrauterine system (LNG-IUS) reduces menstrual blood loss by up to 96%, and 20% of women using the LNG-IUS are reported to be amenorrhoeic after one year.[7] The LNG-IUS also provides very effective contraception. Its effectiveness has been compared to cyclical progestogens, endometrial ablation and hysterectomy. The LNG-IUS is more effective than cyclical norethisterone (for 21 days). The LNG-IUS results in a smaller mean reduction in menstrual blood loss (as assessed by pictorial charts) than endometrial ablation but there is no evidence of a difference in the rate of satisfaction with treatment. Women with an LNG-IUS experience more progestogenic side effects compared to women having endometrial ablation but there is no evidence of a difference in their perceived quality of life. The LNG-IUS treatment costs less than hysterectomy but there is no evidence of a difference in quality of life measures between these groups. However one of the few randomized controlled trials using the LNG-IUS for five years found a 42% hysterectomy rate.[8] The main adverse effect associated with LNG-IUS is frequently occurring variable bleeding and spotting, particularly within the first few months of use. LNG-IUS is also sometimes associated with the development of ovarian cysts, but these are usually symptomless and show a high rate of spontaneous resolution.

The Progestasert® was the first hormonally impregnated device but prospective randomized studies in menorrhagia are lacking.[7] The main disadvantage of this device is its association with an increased risk of ectopic pregnancy.

Oral and intramuscular progestogens

Traditionally, oral progestogen administration was in the luteal phase. However studies with measured menstrual blood loss with luteal administration for seven days of norethisterone 5 mg twice daily show either a decrease or even an increase in flow.[9] However, norethisterone 5 mg three times daily from days 5 to 26 is effective. Side effects include weight gain, headache and bloatedness. Depo-Provera (intramuscular medroxyprogesterone acetate), despite being licensed as a contraceptive, is often used to treat menorrhagia as it can induce amenorrhoea. However, there are no randomized controlled trial data. There are also no data with progestogen-only pills.

Combined oestrogen/progestogen contraceptives

From clinical experience, combined oral contraceptives (COCs) are generally considered to be effective in the management of dysfunctional menstrual bleeding. However, there are few available data to support this observation.[10] There are no data with the contraceptive patch.

Others

Danazol is an isoxazol deivative of 17α-ethinyl-testosterone which acts on the hypothalamic–pituitary axis as well as on the endometrium to produce atrophy. Danazol reduces menstrual blood loss by up to 80% from baseline. Its clinical use is limited by androgenic side effects, which are experienced by up to three-quarters of patients.[4]

Gestrinone is a 19-nortestosterone derivative which has antiprogestogenic, anti-oestrogenic and androgenic activity. In a placebo-controlled study it reduced menstrual blood loss in 79% of patients with objective menorrhagia.[1] However, it also has androgenic side effects.

Gonadotrophin-releasing hormone (GnRH) agonists, administered continuously or in depot form, downregulate expression of GnRH receptors, which blocks gonadotrophin secretion from the anterior pituitary. This leads to ovarian suppression. GnRH agonists have been mainly used in fibroid-associated bleeding.[1] Concerns about the long-term effects of ovarian suppression such as osteoporosis generally limit use beyond six months, even when add-back therapy (oestrogen/progestogen hormone replacement therapy) is used in conjunction.

Recent Developments

1 The LNG-IUS is recommended by the UK National Institute for Health and Clinical Excellence as a first-line treatment provided long-term use (at least 12 months) is anticipated.[4] The use of the LNG-IUS for the management of menorrhagia in primary care (as opposed to women recruited to menorrhagia trials with a menstrual blood loss >80 ml, i.e. objective menorrhagia) is currently being evaluated in the ECLIPSE study (International Standard Randomised Controlled Trial Number 86566246).

2 The United States Food and Drug Administration (FDA) has recently approved the marketing of a monophasic levonorgestrel and ethinyl oestradiol COC in an extended regimen (Seasonale). A patient considered for this regimen would have to be assessed as to whether she had contraindications to COC use such as smoking. One could also consider continuous use without a break. However, neither regimen has been studied in menorrhagia.

Conclusion

Menorrhagia is a common condition. It is important that healthcare professionals should be aware that it is the woman herself who determines whether a treatment is successful for her. What is the first-line treatment for an individual depends on her contraceptive needs. If this woman's family were complete, one would suggest trying the LNG-IUS. This will also provide effective contraception.

Further Reading

1 Oehler MK, Rees MC. Menorrhagia: an update. *Acta Obstet Gynecol Scand* 2003; **82**: 405–22.

2 CKS. Clinical topic. Menorrhagia (heavy menstrual bleeding). www.cks.library.nhs.uk/menorrhagia (accessed 20 09 07)

3 Reid PC, Mukri F. Trends in number of hysterectomies performed in England for menorrhagia: examination of health episode statistics, 1989 to 2002–3. *BMJ* 2005; **330**: 938–9.

4   National Institute for Health and Clinical Excellence. Heavy menstrual bleeding: investigation and treatment. Clinical guideline 44. London: NICE, January 2007. www.nice.org.uk/guidance/CG44 (accessed 20 09 07)

5   Lethaby A, Augood C, Duckitt K. Nonsteroidal anti-inflammatory drugs for heavy menstrual bleeding. *Cochrane Database Syst Rev* 2007; CD000400.

6   Lethaby A, Farquhar C, Cooke I. Antifibrinolytics for heavy menstrual bleeding. *Cochrane Database Syst Rev* 2007; CD000249.

7   Lethaby AE, Cooke I, Rees M. Progesterone or progestogen-releasing intrauterine systems for heavy menstrual bleeding. *Cochrane Database Syst Rev* 2005; CD002126.

8   Hurskainen R, Teperi J, Rissanen P, Aalto AM, Grenman S, Kivelä A, Kujansuu E, Vuorma S, Yliskoski M, Paavonen J. Clinical outcomes and costs with the levonorgestrel-releasing intrauterine system or hysterectomy for treatment of menorrhagia: randomized trial 5-year follow-up. *JAMA* 2004; **291**: 1456–63.

9   Lethaby A, Irvine G, Cameron I. Cyclical progestogens for heavy menstrual bleeding. *Cochrane Database Syst Rev* 2007; CD001016.

10 Davis A, Godwin A, Lippman J, Olson W, Kafrissen M. Triphasic norgestimate-ethinyl estradiol for treating dysfunctional uterine bleeding. *Obstet Gynecol* 2000; **96**: 913–20.

PROBLEM

02 Menorrhagia with Surgical Management

Case History

A 43-year-old woman comes demanding surgical treatment for her menorrhagia. She has tried mefenamic acid and tranexamic acid and her levonorgestrel-releasing intrauterine device has fallen out with a particularly heavy bleed. Her family is complete. She has already been investigated and has no significant pelvic pathology. She cannot cope with the embarrassing flooding and has already ruined a white sofa.

What endometrial ablative techniques can you offer?

How is hysterectomy performed?

How do the different methods compare?

What is life after hysterectomy?

Background

 Surgery is a more definitive treatment for menorrhagia and is appropriate for those in whom medical therapy has failed and whose families are complete.[1,2]

What endometrial ablative techniques can you offer?

Endometrial ablation (EA) aims to destroy the endometrium along with the superficial myometrium thus reducing endometrial shedding at menstruation and resulting in less bleeding.[3] Not all women are amenorrhoeic, with rates varying between 15% and 50%. Directed ablation/resection deals with removal of individual fibroids and polyps. Endometrial ablative techniques are often done as day cases, and a return to normal activities is usually possible within 3–4 days. There are two types of techniques: first generation requiring hysteroscopy, and second generation that do not (Table 2.1). The former are technically more difficult than the latter.

Table 2.1 Methods of endometrial ablation
First generation
Transcervical resection of the endometrium (TCRE)
Endometrial laser ablation (ELA)
Rollerball endometrial ablation (REA)
Second generation
Thermal balloons
Microwave endometrial ablation (MEA)
Circulating hot saline
Cryotherapy

Transcervical endometrial resection (TCRE) involves diathermic removal of the endometrium in strips, similar to a transurethral resection of the prostate. It has been exhaustively proven to be effective. It is the only ablative procedure that obtains endometrial material from the whole of the uterine cavity other than the cornual regions. This may suggest TCRE is more appropriate in peri-menopausal women who have a higher risk of endometrial cancer, though no evidence is available at present to substantiate this theory.

Pre-operative use of endometrial thinning agents, such as danazol or gonadotrophin-releasing hormone analogues, to improve success rates has been recommended for first-generation endometrial ablative techniques where optimum visualization of the cavity is required.

The complications of TCRE have been well documented. These include haemorrhage (2.38%–3.5%), perforation (1%) and fluid overload (0.5%–4%) similar to other first-generation methods of EA such as laser and rollerball endometrial ablation.

Second-generation methods require less operating time and bypass well-recognized first-generation complications by not using fluid with cutting apparatus. In some methods endometrial preparation is also not required, reducing costs and side effects. Although the thermal balloon method is reported to have few complications, it is currently restricted to normal uterine cavities. In comparison, microwave endometrial ablation (MEA) can treat women with irregular uterine cavities in a similar way to TCRE.

In a comparison of the newer non-hysteroscopic techniques (second generation) with the gold-standard hysteroscopic ablative techniques (first generation), surgery was an average of 15 minutes shorter and local anaesthesia was more likely to be employed. Women undergoing newer ablative procedures were less likely to have fluid overload, uterine perforation, cervical lacerations and haematomata than women undergoing the more traditional type of ablation and resection techniques. However there was a higher probability of equipment failure with second-generation ablation techniques.

The main disadvantage of the second-generation endometrial ablative techniques is lack of endometrial material for histology. Although endometrial biopsy is essential prior to all ablations (or a strip of endometrium taken off pre-rollerball), this does not sample the whole uterine cavity and focal endometrial cancer or atypical hyperplasia can be missed.

How is hysterectomy performed?

Hysterectomy is the second most common major operation performed after Caesarean section in the Western world. Hysterectomy appears to be a more definitive operation than EA (Table 2.2), with women undergoing a hysterectomy being less likely to be re-admitted to hospital up to five years after their operation and significantly less likely to be re-admitted for reasons related to their operation, particularly for gynaecological reasons.[4] The three choices are abdominal, vaginal or laparoscopic hysterectomy.[5] Laparoscopic hysterectomy has three further subdivisions: laparoscopic-assisted vaginal hysterectomy, where a vaginal hysterectomy is completed with varying degrees of laparoscopic assistance; subtotal laparoscopic hysterectomy, where the uterine body is removed leaving the cervix in place; and total laparoscopic hysterectomy, where the uterus and cervix are removed and the vaginal vault is sutured laparoscopically. Total abdominal hysterectomy is useful in women with large uteri, fibroid uteri, adenomyosis, endometriosis and pelvic adhesions. Oophorectomy performed at the time of hysterectomy to reduce the risk of ovarian cancer is a controversial issue. In women at low risk and whose ovaries are healthy it is generally advised to retain the ovaries.

There is currently a vogue for subtotal hysterectomy conserving the cervix, with the understanding that sexual function is better preserved than with total hysterectomy. However this has not been confirmed with prospective studies. The downside is that cervical smears have to be continued. Also there may be some endometrium in the cervical stump and this has been reported in 7% of women.[6]

Table 2.2 Comparison of endometrial ablation and hysterectomy		
Issues	Hysterectomy	Endometrial ablation
Amenorrhoea	100% if total	15%–50%
Contraception	Provided	Not provided
Cervical smears	No need unless subtotal	Need to continue
Hormone replacement therapy	Oestrogen only	Oestrogen plus progestogen
Fertility	Offered only if no fertility goals	Offered only if no fertility goals

How do the different methods of hysterectomy compare?

The United Kingdom VALUE study examined complications after hysterectomy.[7] The overall operative complication rate was 3.5%, and highest for the laparoscopic techniques. The overall post-operative complication rate was 9%. One per cent of these were regarded as severe, with the highest rate for severe in the laparoscopic group (2%). There were no operative deaths; 14 deaths were reported within the six-week post-operative period, a crude mortality rate soon after surgery of 0.38 per thousand (95% confidence interval 0.25–0.64). In the international eVALuate study, two parallel multicentre trials compared laparoscopic hysterectomy with abdominal hysterectomy, and laparoscopic hysterectomy with vaginal hysterectomy.[8] Laparoscopic hysterectomy was associated with a higher rate of major complications than abdominal hysterectomy (11.1% vs 6.2%). Laparoscopic hysterectomy also took longer to perform (84 minutes vs 50 minutes) but was less painful and resulted in a shorter stay in hospital after the operation (three days vs four days). There was no evidence of a difference in major complication rates between laparoscopic hysterectomy and vaginal hysterectomy (9.8% vs 9.5%). Again, laparoscopic hysterectomy took longer to perform than vaginal hysterectomy (72 minutes vs 39 minutes).

What is life after hysterectomy?

In the late 1970s it was believed from retrospective studies that hysterectomy increased psychiatric morbidity. Several prospective studies undertaken in the 1980s found a reduction of morbidity six months after surgery. This has been confirmed in a recent study of total versus subtotal hysterectomy.[9] All women showed an improvement in psychological symptoms following both operations and no difference was found between the two procedures.

Early ovarian failure may occur even if ovaries are conserved. These women will require oestrogen-only hormone replacement therapy (HRT). In women who have had a subtotal hysterectomy there may be a concern that there is a remnant of endometrium in the cervical stump.[6] If this is the case, empirically the presence or absence of bleeding induced by monthly sequential HRT may be a useful diagnostic test. If withdrawal bleeds occur, the woman will need oestrogen–progestogen combined HRT. If not, she can have oestrogen-only HRT.

Recent Developments

1 A systematic review found that the benefits of vaginal versus abdominal hysterectomy were shorter duration of hospital stay, speedier return to normal activities and fewer unspecified infections or febrile episodes.[5] The benefits of laparoscopic versus abdominal hysterectomy were lower intra-operative blood loss, shorter duration of hospital stay, speedier return to normal activities, fewer wound or abdominal wall infections and fewer unspecified infections or febrile episodes, at the cost of longer operating time and more urinary tract (bladder or ureter) injuries. There was no evidence of benefits of laparoscopic versus vaginal hysterectomy and the operating time was increased. The authors concluded that vaginal hysterectomy should be performed in preference to abdominal hysterectomy where possible.

2 In the UK, the National Institute for Health and Clinical Excellence states that endometrial ablation may be offered as an initial treatment for menorrhagia after full discussion with the woman of the risks and benefits and of other treatment options.[1] Women must be advised to avoid subsequent pregnancy and on the need to use effective contraception, if required, after endometrial ablation. Hysterectomy should not be used as a first-line treatment solely for menorrhagia. Hysterectomy should be considered only when:

- other treatment options have failed, are contraindicated or are declined by the woman;
- there is a wish for amenorrhoea;
- the woman (who has been fully informed) requests it;
- the woman no longer wishes to retain her uterus and fertility.

Conclusion

 This patient has not responded to medical treatment and her family is complete. She elects to have an endometrial ablation.

Further Reading

1 National Institute for Health and Clinical Excellence. Heavy menstrual bleeding: investigation and treatment. Clinical guideline 44. London: NICE, January 2007. www.nice.org.uk/guidance/CG44 (accessed 20 09 07)

2 CKS. Clinical topic. Menorrhagia (heavy menstrual bleeding). www.cks.library.nhs.uk/menorrhagia (accessed 20 09 07)

3 Lethaby A, Hickey M, Garry R. Endometrial destruction techniques for heavy menstrual bleeding. *Cochrane Database Syst Rev* 2005; CD001501.

4 Clarke A, Judge A, Herbert A, McPherson K, Bridgman S, Maresh M, Overton C, Altman D. Readmission to hospital 5 years after hysterectomy or endometrial resection in a national cohort study. *Qual Saf Health Care* 2005; **14**: 41–7.

5 Johnson N, Barlow D, Lethaby A, Tavender E, Curr E, Garry R. Surgical approach to hysterectomy for benign gynaecological disease. *Cochrane Database Syst Rev* 2006; CD003677.

6 Thakar R, Ayers S, Clarkson P, Stanton S, Manyonda I. Outcomes after total versus subtotal abdominal hysterectomy. *N Engl J Med* 2002; **347**: 1318–25.

7 Maresh MJ, Metcalfe MA, McPherson K, Overton C, Hall V, Hargreaves J, Bridgman S, Dobbins J, Casbard A. The VALUE national hysterectomy study: description of the patients and their surgery. *BJOG* 2002; **109**: 302–12.

8 Garry R, Fountain J, Mason S, Hawe J, Napp V, Abbott J, Clayton R, Phillips G, Whittaker M, Lilford R, Bridgman S, Brown J. The eVALuate study: two parallel randomised trials, one comparing laparoscopic with abdominal hysterectomy, the other comparing laparoscopic with vaginal hysterectomy. *BMJ* 2004; **328**: 129.

9 Thakar R, Ayers S, Georgakapolou A, Clarkson P, Stanton S, Manyonda I. Hysterectomy improves quality of life and decreases psychiatric symptoms: a prospective and randomised comparison of total versus subtotal hysterectomy. *BJOG* 2004; **111**: 1115–20.

03 Dysmenorrhoea

Case History

A 15-year-old girl attends with her mother asking for treatment for her painful periods. She has to take at least one day a month off school because of the pain and is concerned about how this will affect her examination results. She is not yet sexually active.

What specific areas should you explore in the history?

Is a pelvic examination indicated?

What first-line treatments would you recommend?

What non-pharmacological treatments exist?

Is surgery ever indicated?

Background

Dysmenorrhoea is defined as painful menstrual cramps and has been traditionally sub-divided into primary (without any pathology) and secondary dysmenorrhoea (due to other pathology). It is very common, with estimates of prevalence ranging from 20% to 90%.[1] Most adolescents self-medicate rather than consult a doctor; however, dysmenorrhoea is the most common cause of recurrent school absenteeism in teenage girls. It is important, therefore, that it is identified and treated early.

What specific areas should you explore in the history?

Pain with menstruation will usually commence within a year of menarche, thus if it starts beyond this period it should alert to the possibility of other pathology (such as endometriosis or adenomyosis).[2] Therefore, age at menarche and age at which dysmenorrhoea began should be elicited. An attempt should be made to understand the bleeding pattern, as initial anovulatory cycles are often more irregular, heavier and more painful and this may improve as cycles become ovulatory and more regular. Associated symptoms may include radiation of pain to the back or thighs, nausea, vomiting or diarrhoea. However, cyclical rectal bleeding or other bowel symptoms may point to a diagnosis of rectal endometriosis or irritable bowel syndrome. The pain usually starts no more than a few hours before the onset of menstruation and settles after the first 24–36 hours. More prolonged pain or pain of a non-cyclical nature should raise the suspicion of other pathology. Dysmenorrhoea usually improves after childbirth and if parity is controlled for there is no relationship with age.[3] However, depression and anxiety, disruption of social networks and smoking are all associated factors.[1] As many of the initial treatments are available over the counter, what treatments have been tried and whether or not they were successful at all should be established.

Is a pelvic examination indicated?

As long as nothing in the history suggests another pathology, there is no need for a pelvic examination prior to commencing empirical treatment, especially in girls who are not yet sexually active. Abnormal vaginal discharge or risk of sexually transmitted infections should prompt internal examination and appropriate swabs.

What first-line treatments would you recommend?

Dysmenorrhoea is thought to be due to increased prostaglandin production by the endometrium which causes stronger and more irregular uterine contractions, reducing uterine blood flow and causing painful, transient ischaemia. Prostaglandins are also likely to be responsible for the nausea, vomiting and diarrhoea which are often associated with the pain.[2] Thus first-line medical treatment is usually non-steroidal anti-inflammatory drugs (NSAIDs), such as ibuprofen and naproxen sodium, because of their action in reducing prostaglandin synthesis as well as a central analgesic action.[4] In order for them to be effective they need to be commenced at or just before the onset of menstruation and continued at regular intervals throughout the first two days, rather than waiting for the pain to increase. Their half-life is a few hours. NSAIDs have been shown to be significantly more effective at relieving dysmenorrhoea when compared to placebo, but there is insufficient evidence to recommend any one drug over another.[5] NSAIDs are not without side effects; however, if just taken for two days a month by otherwise healthy girls or women they are likely to be well tolerated. More recently, cyclooxygenase-2 (COX-2)-specific inhibitors have been shown to be similarly efficacious.[6] However, there are current safety concerns and thus they cannot be recommended over traditional NSAIDs.

Combined oral contraceptive pills induce endometrial atrophy and thus reduce menstrual fluid prostaglandins as well as reducing the amount of bleeding and pain. They are therefore also recommended as a first-line treatment, especially if contraception is required. Although they are effective clinically, the studies are small and of poor quality.[7] It would be prudent, however, to check whether contraception is needed and see the patient alone without her mother.

What non-pharmacological treatments exist?

A number of dietary supplements and modifications have been suggested to improve dysmenorrhoea, although convincing evidence does not exist for most of these in humans. Both fish oil and krill oil, however, were shown to have a significant effect.[2,4] Transcutaneous electrical nerve stimulation has been shown to be effective in both reducing dysmenorrhoea and reducing analgesia usage,[8] as has continuous low-level topical heat,[9] although neither of these are as easy to manage outside the home as simple analgesics. There is limited evidence that exercise reduces dysmenorrhoea.[2]

Is surgery ever indicated?

If dysmenorrhoea does not respond to first-line treatments then a laparoscopy may be justified to look for other causes of pain such as endometriosis or congenital uterine abnormalities. Ultrasound and magnetic resonance imaging (MRI) scans pre-operatively may also help investigate the pain.

A few studies have looked at the role of laparoscopic uterine nerve ablation (LUNA) and presacral neurectomy (PSN) in women whose dysmenorrhoea is severe and refractory to other treatments. PSN appears to be effective in a small number of women whereas LUNA is not; however, the long-term benefits are not known.[10]

Recent Developments

Behavioural interventions for dysmenorrhoea have been examined in a systematic review.[11] Five trials involving 213 women were included. Behavioural intervention vs control: One trial of pain management training reported reduction in pain and symptoms compared to a control. Three trials of relaxation compared to control reported varied results, two trials showed no difference in symptom severity scores, however one trial reported that relaxation was effective for reducing symptoms in menstrual sufferers with spasmodic symptoms. Two trials reported less restriction in daily activities following treatment with either relaxation or pain management training compared to a control. One trial also reported less time absent from school following treatment with pain management training compared to a control. The authors concluded that there is some evidence from five RCTs that behavioural interventions may be effective for dysmenorrhoea, however results should be viewed with caution as they varied greatly between trials due to inconsistency in the reporting of data, small trial size, poor methodological quality and age of the trials.

Conclusion

It is essential that this patient is taken seriously. The pathophysiology of dysmenorrhoea needs to be explained and effective treatment instigated. If appropriate, further investigations should be undertaken, but many patients can be effectively managed with simple analgesics or the combined oral contraceptive pill.

Further Reading

1 French L. Dysmenorrhea. *Am Fam Physician* 2005; **71**: 285–91.

2 Dawood MY. Primary dysmenorrhea: advances in pathogenesis and management. *Obstet Gynecol* 2006; **108**: 428–41.

3 Sundell G, Milsom I, Andersch B. Factors influencing the prevalence and severity of dysmenorrhoea in young women. *Br J Obstet Gynaecol* 1990; **97**: 588–94.

4 Proctor M, Farquhar C. Diagnosis and management of dysmenorrhoea. *BMJ* 2006; **332**: 1134–8.

5 Marjoribanks J, Proctor ML, Farquhar C. Nonsteroidal anti-inflammatory drugs for primary dysmenorrhoea. *Cochrane Database Syst Rev* 2003; CD001751.

6 Daniels SE, Talwalker S, Torri S, Snabes MC, Recker DP, Verburg KM. Valdecoxib, a cyclooxygenase-2-specific inhibitor, is effective in treating primary dysmenorrhea. *Obstet Gynecol* 2002; **100**: 350–8.

7 Proctor ML, Roberts H, Farquhar CM. Combined oral contraceptive pill (OCP) as treatment for primary dysmenorrhoea. *Cochrane Database Syst Rev* 2001; CD002120.

8 Proctor ML, Smith CA, Farquhar CM, Stones RW. Transcutaneous electrical nerve stimulation and acupuncture for primary dysmenorrhoea. *Cochrane Database Syst Rev* 2002; CD002123.

9 Akin MD, Weingand KW, Hengehold DA, Goodale MB, Hinkle RT, Smith RP. Continuous low-level topical heat in the treatment of dysmenorrhea. *Obstet Gynecol* 2001; **97**: 343–9.

10 Proctor M, Latthe P, Farquhar C, Khan KS, Johnson N. Surgical interruption of pelvic nerve pathways for primary and secondary dysmenorrhoea. *Cochrane Database Syst Rev* 2005; CD001896.

11 Proctor M, Murphy P, Pattison H, Suckling J, Farquhar C. Behavioural interventions for primary and secondary dysmenorrhoea. *Cochrane Database Syst Rev* 2007; CD002248.

PROBLEM

04 Chronic Pelvic Pain

Case History

A 32-year-old woman presents with a ten-year history of pelvic pain which is present most days of the month but has cyclical exacerbations. She is nulliparous, although she underwent a surgical termination of pregnancy (TOP) at age 17 years. Currently she is not in a stable relationship. Previously she had two diagnostic laparoscopies, both of which were completely normal.

What areas should you explore in the history?

What are you looking for on examination?

Are any investigations justified?

What treatment might be appropriate?

Background

 Chronic pelvic pain (CPP) is a symptom not a diagnosis and is defined as 'intermittent or constant pain in the lower abdomen or pelvis of at least six months' duration, not occurring exclusively with menstruation or intercourse and not associated with pregnancy'.[1] It has been shown to have an annual prevalence of 38/1000 in women aged 15–73 years old, which is comparable to asthma (37/100) and back pain (41/1000).[2] A number of studies have shown that many women (e.g. 25% after 3–4 years follow-up in one study) receive no diagnostic label even after multiple invasive investigations and many years.[2] The symptom of CPP can be caused by pathology in a number of organ systems which overlap many specialities, contributing to diagnostic delay (see Table 4.1). Furthermore, more than one pathology can coexist and psychological factors also alter the experience of the pain. It has been shown that women with CPP have an increased incidence of negative cognitive features and emotional traits; however, it is not possible to ascertain whether these are involved in generating the chronic pain state or if they are a consequence of living with the pain and frequent attempts to justify its reality or severity to health professionals.[3] A number of factors have been identified which predispose women to developing CPP,[4] although the symptom occurs across all socio-economic groups. It has been shown that women want validation of their symptoms and reassurance from the consultation[5] and therefore taking a history alone can be therapeutic.

Table 4.1 Possible contributory factors in CPP

Gynaecological	Gastrointestinal	Urinary	Musculoskeletal	Psychological
Endometriosis	Inflammatory bowel disease	Interstitial cystitis	Fibromyalgia	Depression
Adenomyosis	Irritable bowel disease	Urethral syndrome	Disc disease	Physical/sexual abuse
Chronic pelvic inflammatory disease		Calculi	Hernia	Somatization
Adhesions			Arthritis	
Residual ovarian syndrome			Sacroiliac joint dysfunction	
Trapped ovary syndrome			Piriformis syndrome	

What areas should you explore in the history?

A detailed history of the pain should be taken; however, it may be necessary to suggest to the woman that she keeps a detailed pain diary over the next one to two cycles so that patterns can be identified. The nature, location and radiation of the pain are important. Sharp stabbing or aching, burning pain may suggest neuropathic pain. Bowel and bladder function should also be discussed in detail as irritable bowel syndrome (IBS) and interstitial cystitis (IC) can both have a cyclical pattern. Dyspareunia should be addressed as its presence may help with the diagnosis and it has a negative effect on quality of life for the woman.

As the pain has been present for a number of years, events preceding/surrounding the onset of the pain may be difficult to recall, but this area should be explored as well as the woman's emotions surrounding her TOP. This could lead into a discussion of future fertility plans as there are often concerns that a TOP could have caused long-lasting damage which could affect fertility. It is important to elicit the woman's own beliefs and concerns about what is causing her pain. A history of abuse has been linked to CPP and this area should be explored if it is appropriate; however, this is often not possible at the first appointment.

What are you looking for on examination?

The purpose of the examination is twofold. It should give clues towards the diagnosis, and it is also the time the woman is at her most vulnerable, and during an internal examination, particularly, new information is often revealed.[6]

Abdominal palpation may reveal a musculoskeletal cause for the pain, or a trigger point (a discrete, focal, hyperirritable spot in a taut band of skeletal muscle) may be identified[7] which can be injected with local anaesthetic. Altered sensation in the skin may also be noted. Internal examination may demonstrate the presence of vaginismus or hypercontractility of the pelvic floor which may respond to physiotherapy. Uterosacral tenderness or nodules may be palpable as may other pelvic pathology such as uterine tenderness or ovarian cysts. An abnormal discharge should also be looked for.

Are any investigations justified?

Traditionally a laparoscopy has been performed to investigate pelvic pain. However, this procedure in itself is not without risk (2/1000 risk of serious complications, 3–8/100 000 risk of death)[8] and not all causes of CPP will be visible at laparoscopy (e.g. IBS, adenomyosis). There are also concerns that deeply infiltrating endometriosis may also be missed at laparoscopy. Therefore it may not be the most appropriate first-line investigation,[1] especially if there are other risk factors present such as an increased body mass index, previous laparotomy, etc. It was previously thought that showing a woman photographs of her pelvis after a negative laparoscopy would improve her pain; however, studies have shown this not to be true,[9] and it may actually reinforce her beliefs that her pain is not taken seriously or thought to be in her head.

If there are concerns about infection then swabs may be indicated, although referral to a genitourinary medicine clinic is often more appropriate. A magnetic resonance imaging (MRI) scan can be useful to show deeply infiltrating endometriosis or adenomyosis. If fertility is a concern, a laparoscopy may be appropriate to test tubal patency and treat any adhesions or endometriosis. Reassurance about fertility may reduce the pain experience considerably.

What treatment might be appropriate?

Treatment needs to be tailored to the specific patient, her predominant symptoms and current and future fertility desires (Figure 4.1). As there is a cyclical component to the pain, hormonal treatment may be appropriate. This could be in the form of the combined oral contraceptive pill (taken conventionally, tricycling or continuously), a gonadotrophin-releasing hormone (GnRH) agonist or the levonorgestrel intrauterine system (LNG-IUS) coil. If a good response is obtained with a GnRH agonist and the woman would like to continue with this form of treatment, there is now evidence to suggest that as long as low-dose hormone replacement therapy is given as well, treatment can be safely continued for at least two years,[10] if not ten.[11] Both IBS and IC have been shown to respond in some instances to hormonal treatment. Otherwise, alteration of diet plus the use of regular fibre supplementation and referral to a dietician or gastroenterologist in the case of IBS may be necessary.

Particularly where musculoskeletal or pelvic floor abnormalities are identified, referral to a physiotherapist may be helpful. If the woman acknowledges that psychological issues play a part in her pain or worsen the pain experience then referral to a counsellor may be appropriate; however, this suggestion may have to be broached gently if she has been repeatedly told that her pain is in her head.

Finally, if there is a neuropathic element to the pain, treatment with amitriptyline, gabapentin or pregabalin could help. A number of these strategies can be commenced together as a multidisciplinary approach is often most successful.

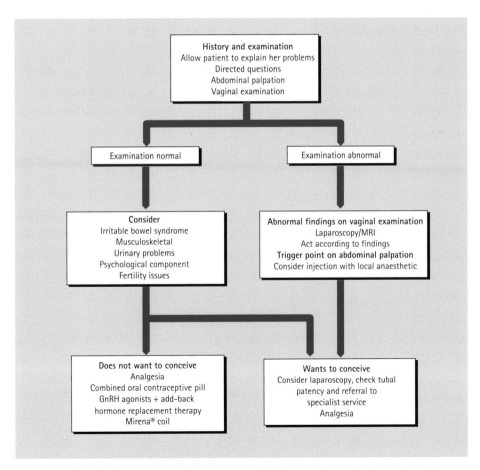

Figure 4.1 Algorithm for the suggested management of CPP. *Source:* adapted from Kennedy and Moore 2005.[1]

Recent Developments

As the understanding of the complex nature of pelvic pain has developed, interest has focused on the role of the central nervous system in pain modulation.[12,13] Musculoskeletal abnormalities and neuropathies are increasingly recognized as relevant. Trigger point injections may be effective.[12]

Conclusion

Chronic pelvic pain is common. It is a symptom rather than a diagnosis in itself and much remains unclear about its aetiology. Treatment needs to be tailored to the patient. A number of strategies can be commenced together as a multidisciplinary approach is often most successful.

Further Reading

1 Royal College of Obstetricians and Gynaecologists (RCOG). The initial management of chronic pelvic pain. Green-top Guideline No. 41. London: RCOG Press, 2005.

2 Zondervan KT, Yudkin PL, Vessey MP, Dawes MG, Barlow DH, Kennedy SH. Prevalence and incidence of chronic pelvic pain in primary care: evidence from a national general practice database. *Br J Obstet Gynaecol* 1999; **106**: 1149–55.

3 Newton-John T. The psychology of pain. In: MacLean A, Stones RW, Thornton S (eds). *Pain in Obstetrics and Gynaecology*. London: RCOG Press, 2001; 59–69.

4 Latthe P, Mignini L, Gray R, Hills R, Khan K. Factors predisposing women to chronic pelvic pain: systematic review. *BMJ* 2006; **332**: 749–55.

5 Price J, Farmer G, Harris J, Hope T, Kennedy S, Mayou R. Attitudes of women with chronic pelvic pain to the gynaecological consultation: a qualitative study. *BJOG* 2006; **113**: 446–52.

6 Skrine R, Mountford H (eds). *Psychosexual Medicine: An Introduction*. London: Arnold, 2001.

7 Prendergast SA, Weiss J. Screening for musculoskeletal causes of pelvic pain. *Clin Obstet Gynecol* 2003; **46**: 773–82.

8 Chapron C, Querleu D, Bruhat MA, Madelenat P, Fernandez H, Pierre F, Dubuisson JB. Surgical complications of diagnostic and operative gynaecological laparoscopy: a series of 29,966 cases. *Hum Reprod* 1998; **13**: 867–72.

9 Onwude JL, Thornton JG, Morley S, Lilleymen J, Currie I, Lilford RJ. A randomised trial of photographic reinforcement during postoperative counselling after diagnostic laparoscopy for pelvic pain. *Eur J Obstet Gynecol Reprod Biol* 2004; **112**: 89–94.

10 Sagsveen M, Farmer JE, Prentice A, Breeze A. Gonadotrophin-releasing hormone analogues for endometriosis: bone mineral density. *Cochrane Database Syst Rev* 2003; CD001297.

11 Bedaiwy MA, Casper RF. Treatment with leuprolide acetate and hormonal add-back for up to 10 years in stage IV endometriosis patients with chronic pelvic pain. *Fertil Steril* 2006; **86**: 220–2.

12 Langford CF, Udvari Nagy S, Ghoniem GM. Levator ani trigger point injections: An underutilized treatment for chronic pelvic pain. *Neurourol Urodyn* 2007; **26**: 59–62.

13 Bingel U, Schoell E, Buchel C. Imaging pain modulation in health and disease. *Curr Opin Neurol* 2007; **20**: 424–31

PROBLEM

05 Endometriosis

Case History

A 27-year-old woman presents with an 18-month history of pelvic pain, dyspareunia and failure to conceive despite regular intercourse. Four years earlier a laparoscopy had confirmed endometriosis which was ablated and she was pain-free whilst tricycling the combined oral contraceptive (COC) pill.

What are the first-line treatments for pain associated with endometriosis?

Is a diagnostic laparoscopy necessary before commencing treatment?

How should treatment differ if pain is present and the woman is trying to conceive?

If an endometrioma was found on ultrasound scan, how should this be managed?

Background

Endometriosis is defined as 'the presence of endometrial-like tissue outside the uterus, which induces a chronic, inflammatory reaction'. It is common; however, the exact prevalence is not known as not every woman has a laparoscopy in order to look for disease. There is still debate about aetiology, but it is likely to be a combination of retrograde menstruation[1] and an altered immune environment which allows the ectopic tissue to implant and develop a blood and nerve supply.[2] Clinical presentation can be very variable and correlates poorly with the extent of disease seen at laparoscopy.[3] Treatment needs to be tailored to the woman's particular symptoms, her age and her reproductive wishes, both current and future.

What are the first-line treatments for pain associated with endometriosis?

Simple analgesics, such as non-steroidal anti-inflammatory drugs (NSAIDs), have traditionally been first-line treatments for endometriosis. However, a meta-analysis found that only one randomized controlled trial was considered robust enough to be included, and there was no evidence of a positive effect on pain relief when comparing naproxen to placebo in women with endometriosis.[4] If women are avoiding hormonal treatment because of a desire for pregnancy, they need to be aware that NSAIDs have an anti-ovulatory effect when taken mid-cycle, as well as other adverse effects such as gastric ulceration.

A variety of hormonal treatments have also been shown to be successful in reducing the pain associated with endometriosis. These include the COC pill,[5] progestogens,[6] danazol[7] and gonadotrophin-releasing hormone agonists (GnRHa).[8] These have all been shown to be equally effective at reducing pain, but have different side-effect profiles and costs. An intrauterine levonorgestrel-releasing system can also be effective.[1]

Is a diagnostic laparoscopy necessary before commencing treatment?

Current guidelines suggest that pain thought to be due to endometriosis can be treated either with simple analgesia or hormonal treatments without the need for a definitive surgical diagnosis.[9,10] Laparoscopy is the gold standard for making a diagnosis, but is not without risk. Positive histology is not required to confirm the diagnosis; however, if endometriomas greater than 3 cm diameter are found, histology should be obtained.[9]

How should treatment differ if pain is present and the woman is trying to conceive?

Ovarian suppression with hormonal treatments has not been shown to increase pregnancy rates[11] and therefore is not recommended. A laparoscopy should be considered, as adhesions can be divided and endometriosis ablated, which may increase pregnancy rates.[9]

With more severe disease, referral should be made to a specialist centre with the necessary experience. Available evidence suggests that any improvement in fertility occurs immediately post-operatively and declines subsequently, such that women should be encouraged to attempt to conceive or undergo assisted conception treatments as appropriate without delay. Though small studies suggest lower success rates with assisted conception in the presence of endometriosis, this is not seen in large databases.[9]

If an endometrioma was found on ultrasound scan, how should this be managed?

Though there are a number of management options for endometriomas, current evidence suggests that laparoscopic ovarian cystectomy should be performed for endometriomas greater than 4 cm diameter. Such endometriomas are unlikely to resolve with hormonal treatment alone. There is a risk of reduced ovarian function post-operatively; however, removal of the endometrioma facilitates egg collection, reduces the risk of infection during *in vitro* fertilization (IVF) and decreases progression of the disease.[12] If laparoscopic cystectomy is not possible, endometriomas can be drained transvaginally; however, this increases the risk of recurrence (up to 100% in some studies), infection and adhesion formation (Table 5.1).

Table 5.1	Advantages and disadvantages of surgical treatment of endometriomas before IVF cycles

Advantages

Facilitates egg collection

Reduces the risk of infection during IVF

Decreases disease progression

Reduces risk of contamination with endometrioma content

Disadvantages

Reduced ovarian function

Risk of surgery

Surgical damage

No evidence it improves pregnancy rates

Source: adapted from Somigliana *et al.* 2006[12]

Recent Developments

Gonadotrophin-releasing hormone agonists are generally well tolerated, and are effective in relieving the symptoms of endometriosis. However, the induced hypoestrogenic state leads to a loss in bone mineral density thereby increasing the risk of osteoporotic fracture. A systematic review of 15 studies showed that danazol and progesterone + oestrogen add-back are protective of bone mineral density (BMD) at the lumbar spine both during treatment and for up to six and twelve months after treatment, respectively.[13] Between the groups receiving GnRHa and the groups receiving danazol/gestrinone, there was a significant difference in percentage change in BMD after six months of treatment, the GnRH analogue producing a reduction in BMD from baseline and danazol producing an increase in BMD (BMD −3.43; 95% confidence interval [CI] −3.91 to −2.95). Progesterone only add-back was not protective. The authors concluded that both danazol and progesterone + oestrogen add-back were protective of BMD, while on treatment and up to six and twelve months later, respectively. However, by 24 months of follow-up there was no difference in BMD in those women who had hormone replacement therapy (HRT) add-back. Studies of danazol versus GnRHa did not report long-term follow-up. This issue is a major concern since gonadotrophin-releasing hormone agonists have been used for less than 30 years and it is only over the next few decades that their effects on the fracture rate in women over the age of 50 will become clearer.

Conclusion

Endometriosis should be suspected in any woman of reproductive age who presents with dysmenorrhoea or chronic pelvic pain. A common complaint is the delay in diagnosis. Laparoscopy is the gold standard for identifying endometriosis. In women who wish to conceive, surgical rather than medical treatment should be offered.

Further Reading

1 Farquhar C. Endometriosis. *BMJ* 2007; **334**: 249–53.

2 Kyama C, Debrock S, Mwenda J, D'Hooghe T. Potential involvement of the immune system in the development of endometriosis. *Reprod Biol Endocrinol* 2003; **1**: 123.

3 Chapron C, Fauconnier A, Dubuisson JB, Barakat H, Vieira M, Breart G. Deep infiltrating endometriosis: relation between severity of dysmenorrhoea and extent of disease. *Hum Reprod* 2003; **18**: 760–6.

4 Allen C, Hopewell S, Prentice A. Non-steroidal anti-inflammatory drugs for pain in women with endometriosis. *Cochrane Database Syst Rev* 2005; CD004753.

5 Davis L, Kennedy S, Moore J, Prentice A. Modern combined oral contraceptives for pain associated with endometriosis. *Cochrane Database Syst Rev* 2007; CD001019.

6 Prentice A, Deary AJ, Bland E. Progestagens and anti-progestagens for pain associated with endometriosis. *Cochrane Database Syst Rev* 2000; CD002122.

7 Selak V, Farquhar C, Prentice A, Singla A. Danazol for pelvic pain associated with endometriosis. *Cochrane Database Syst Rev* 2001; CD000068.

8 Prentice A, Deary AJ, Goldbeck-Wood S, Farquhar C, Smith SK. Gonadotrophin-releasing hormone analogues for pain associated with endometriosis. *Cochrane Database Syst Rev* 2000; CD000346.

9 Royal College of Obstetricians and Gynaecologists (RCOG). *The Investigation and Management of Endometriosis*. Green-top Guideline No. 24. London: RCOG Press, 2006.

10 Kennedy S, Bergqvist A, Chapron C, D'Hooghe T, Dunselman G, Greb R, Hummelshoj L, Prentice A, Saridogan E. ESHRE guideline for the diagnosis and treatment of endometriosis. *Hum Reprod* 2005; **20**: 2698–704.

11 Hughes E, Brown J, Collins J, Farquhar C, Fedorkow D, Vandekerckhove P. Ovulation suppression for endometriosis. *Cochrane Database Syst Rev* 2007; CD000155.

12 Somigliana E, Vercellini P, Vigano P, Ragni G, Crosignani PG. Should endometriomas be treated before IVF-ICSI cycles? *Hum Reprod Update* 2006; **12**: 57–64.

13 Sagsveen M, Farmer JE, Prentice A, Breeze A. Gonadotrophin-releasing hormone analogues for endometriosis: bone mineral density. *Cochrane Database Syst Rev* 2003; CD001297.

06 Fibroids

Case History

A 39-year-old woman has been found to have four 5 cm diameter fibroids when she had a scan after complaining of bladder irritation and heavier periods. They are mainly intramural but all have a significant subserosal component. She is nulliparous, has no partner and wants to avoid hysterectomy.

What are the medical options?

What are the surgical options?

What are the benefits and risks of uterine artery embolization?

Background

Uterine leiomyomas (fibroids) are benign smooth muscle tumours and are the most common gynaecologic tumours in women of reproductive age.[1,2] Uterine leiomyomas clinically affect 25%–30% of American women; however, an incidence of upwards of 77% has been reported.[1,2] They are more common in African-American women, with some studies indicating they are diagnosed three times more frequently than in white women.[1,2] They are often associated with reproductive and gynaecologic disorders ranging from infertility and pregnancy loss, to pelvic pain, and excessive uterine bleeding. They are steroid-dependent tumours that rarely progress to malignancy and regress at the menopause.

What are the medical options?

The aim of the medical options is to reduce her menstrual bleeding and to reduce fibroid size. With regard to the former, medical options will not improve her pressure symptoms. Options to reduce fibroid size tend to be of limited value and the fibroids will regrow when treatment is stopped.

Non-steroidal anti-inflammatory drugs and antifibrinolytic agents

Non-steroidal anti-inflammatory drugs (NSAIDs) and antifibrinolytic agents are used to reduce menstrual blood loss (see Case 1: Menorrhagia with Medical Management). However, they may be less effective in the presence of fibroids, especially if they are submucous fibroids.

Medroxyprogesterone acetate

Depot medroxyprogesterone acetate in case–controlled studies is associated with a protective effect on the development of fibroids. Clinical trial data in the management of fibroids are limited. A six-month clinical trial of 20 women found that 30% became amenorrhoeic and 70% noticed improvement in their bleeding pattern.[3] Mean uterine and fibroid volume was also reduced by 48% and 33%, respectively.

Intrauterine levonorgestrel

Intrauterine levonorgestrel (levonorgestrel intrauterine system [LNG-IUS]) is a very effective treatment for menorrhagia but there are comparatively few studies in women with fibroids. Expulsion rate may be higher in women with a cavity distorted by fibroids. A systematic review found that all studies directly assessing LNG-IUS in women with fibroids reported decreased menstrual blood loss (84%–90%) and similar increases in haemoglobin of 2–3 g/dl.[4] However, there was inconsistency on whether LNG-IUS is associated with decreased fibroid or no change in fibroid size.

Gonadotrophin-releasing hormone (GnRH) analogues

GnRH analogues produce amenorrhoea and fibroid shrinkage. Unfortunately, shrinkage is rarely complete and not sustained after cessation of therapy. Another concern is the bone mineral loss due to the induced hypo-oestrogenic state limiting use to six months. If given prior to surgery, they can reduce intra-operative blood loss and enable either a Pfannenstiel's incision or a vaginal hysterectomy to be performed. They have been used prior to myomectomy, although experience is relatively limited, but the procedure of enucleation does not appear to be enhanced and blood loss is not reduced. Add-back therapy with oestrogen/progestogen or tibolone has been used to counteract the adverse skeletal effects and this does not seem to adversely affect fibroid shrinkage.[2]

Progesterone receptor antagonists and selective progesterone receptor modulators (SPRMs)

The progesterone receptor antagonist mifepristone has been found to reduce fibroid volume in a limited number of studies, but there are concerns about the development of endometrial hyperplasia.[2,5]

Limited data suggest that raloxifene, used in the treatment of post-menopausal osteoporosis, can shrink fibroids.[6]

What are the surgical options?

Myomectomy is a fertility-sparing procedure but there is the potential for significant haemorrhage that may require hysterectomy as a life-saving procedure. Also there may be significant adhesion formation which may have an adverse effect on fertility. There is also a risk of uterine scar rupture during labour. Myomectomy can be performed either laparoscopically, hysteroscopically or by laparotomy. While recovery is shorter after laparoscopic surgery, this has to be balanced against the longer operating time. There is concern about fibroid recurrence after myomectomy.[7] A five-year study found that cumulative rates for leiomyoma recurrence and subsequent major surgery were 62% and 9%, respectively.[8] At five years, the cumulative probability of recurrence was significantly lower in patients with a single leiomyoma removed (11%) compared with patients with multiple leiomyomata (74%); it was also lower in patients with intra-operative uterine size ten menstrual weeks or less (46%) compared with more than ten menstrual weeks (82%). Childbirth after myomectomy was associated with a lower recurrence rate; the five-year cumulative probability of recurrence was 26% in patients with subsequent parity compared with 76% in those without.

What are the benefits and risks of uterine artery embolization?

Uterine artery embolization (UAE) was first developed as a treatment for massive obstetric haemorrhage. It has been reported to be an effective and safe alternative in the treatment of menorrhagia and other fibroid-related symptoms in women not desiring future fertility.[8] While pregnancies have been reported after UAE, little is known about the long-term effects on the offspring and pregnancy should be avoided. Also, UAE reduces ovarian reserve.[9] Consequently, UAE should not be offered to women wishing to conceive. UAE involves catheterization of the femoral artery. Using angiography to direct a guide wire, a catheter is then passed into the uterine arteries and polyvinyl alcohol (PVA) particles and small pieces of gelatin sponge are used to embolize and occlude the vessels (Figure 6.1). The fibroids then undergo ischaemic necrosis, which is accompanied by a variable amount of pain. About 15% of women will experience post-embolization syndrome with fever, nausea and vomiting. Less common complications are the need for further surgery, such as hysterectomy, and the development of premature ovarian failure, particularly in women aged over 45 years. Rarely, haemorrhage, non-target embolization causing tissue

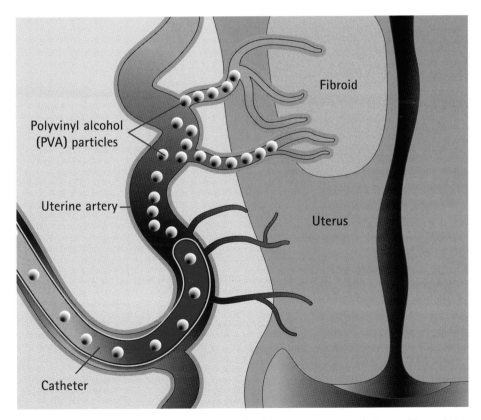

Figure 6.1 Injection of particles of polyvinyl alcohol (PVA) under X-ray guidance (redrawn with permission from Fibroid Medical Center of Northern California, Inc.).

necrosis, and infection causing septicaemia may occur. There will be no histological diagnosis. While fibroids are benign, malignant change can occur, albeit rarely. Little is known about fibroid recurrence after UAE. A systematic review of three trials comparing UAE and hysterectomy or myomectomy found that UAE offers an advantage over hysterectomy with regards to a shorter hospital stay and a quicker return to routine activities.[8] There is no evidence of benefit of UAE compared to surgery (hysterectomy or myomectomy) for satisfaction. The higher minor complications rate after discharge from hospital in the UAE group, as well as the higher unscheduled visits and re-admission rates, require more longer-term follow-up trials to comment on its effectiveness and safety profile. Other subsequent studies have also found shorter recovery times with UAE, with some also reporting a higher need for further intervention in the UAE group.[10–12]

Recent Developments

1 Asoprisnil (J867) is the first SPRM to reach an advanced stage of clinical development for the treatment of symptomatic uterine fibroids and further data are awaited.[13]

2 Myolyis is a technique to destroy fibroids using one of a number of focused energy delivery systems including radiofrequency electricity, supercooled cryoprobes, and focused ultrasound monitored by real-time magnetic resonance imaging.[14,15] Clinical evaluation has been confined to case series, but it is evident that the approach results in a variable degree of reduction of the total uterine mass and, usually, a reduction in uterine bleeding. Clearly, longer-term appropriately designed comparative trials are required.

Conclusion

The options that are acceptable to this woman depend on her fertility goals. Medical options will reduce her symptoms but there are concerns about regrowth when agents such as GnRH analogues are stopped. The long-term effects of UAE remain to be evaluated especially with the risk of early ovarian failure and the need for hormone replacement which may then cause fibroid regrowth.

Further Reading

1 Dixon D, Parrott EC, Segars JH, Olden K, Pinn VW. The second National Institutes of Health International Congress on advances in uterine leiomyoma research: conference summary and future recommendations. *Fertil Steril* 2006; **86**: 800–6.

2 Morrison J, MacKenzie IZ. Uterine fibroids. In: Rees M, Hope S, Ravnikar V (eds). *The Abnormal Menstrual Cycle*. Abingdon: Taylor and Francis, 2005; 79–93.

3 Venkatachalam S, Bagratee JS, Moodley J. Medical management of uterine fibroids with medroxyprogesterone acetate (Depo Provera): a pilot study. *J Obstet Gynaecol* 2004; **24**: 798–800.

4 Varma R, Sinha D, Gupta JK. Non-contraceptive uses of levonorgestrel-releasing hormone system (LNG-IUS) – a systematic enquiry and overview. *Eur J Obstet Gynecol Reprod Biol* 2006; **125**: 9–28.

5 Fiscella K, Eisinger SH, Meldrum S, Feng C, Fisher SG, Guzick DS. Effect of mifepristone for symptomatic leiomyomata on quality of life and uterine size: a randomized controlled trial. *Obstet Gynecol* 2006; **108**: 1381–7.

6 Jirecek S, Lee A, Pavo I, Crans G, Eppel W, Wenzl R. Raloxifene prevents the growth of uterine leiomyomas in premenopausal women. *Fertil Steril* 2004; **81**: 132–6.

7 Hanafi M. Predictors of leiomyoma recurrence after myomectomy. *Obstet Gynecol* 2005; **105**: 877–81.

8 Gupta JK, Sinha AS, Lumsden MA, Hickey M. Uterine artery embolization for symptomatic uterine fibroids. *Cochrane Database Syst Rev* 2006; CD005073.

9 Hehenkamp WJ, Volkers NA, Broekmans FJ, de Jong FH, Themmen AP, Birnie E, Reekers JA, Ankum WM. Loss of ovarian reserve after uterine artery embolization: a randomized comparison with hysterectomy. *Hum Reprod* 2007; **22**: 1996–2005.

10 Edwards RD, Moss JG, Lumsden MA, Wu O, Murray LS, Twaddle S, Murray GD. Uterine-artery embolization versus surgery for symptomatic uterine fibroids. *N Engl J Med* 2007; **356**: 360–70.

11 Volkers NA, Hehenkamp WJ, Birnie E, de Vries C, Holt C, Ankum WM, Reekers JA. Uterine artery embolization in the treatment of symptomatic uterine fibroid tumors (EMMY trial): periprocedural results and complications. *J Vasc Interv Radiol* 2006; **17**: 471–80.

12 Goodwin SC, Bradley LD, Lipman JC, Stewart EA, Nosher JL, Sterling KM, Barth MH, Siskin GP, Shlansky-Goldberg RD. Uterine artery embolization versus myomectomy: a multicenter comparative study. *Fertil Steril* 2006; **85**: 14–21.

13 Chwalisz K, Perez MC, Demanno D, Winkel C, Schubert G, Elger W. Selective progesterone receptor modulator development and use in the treatment of leiomyomata and endometriosis. *Endocr Rev* 2005; **26**: 423–38.

14 Zupi E, Sbracia M, Marconi D, Munro MG. Myolysis of uterine fibroids: is there a role? *Clin Obstet Gynecol* 2006; **49**: 821–33.

15 Smart OC, Hindley JT, Regan L, Gedroyc WG. Gonadotrophin-releasing hormone and magnetic-resonance-guided ultrasound surgery for uterine leiomyomata. *Obstet Gynecol* 2006; **108**: 49–54.

PROBLEM

07 Primary Amenorrhoea

Case History

A 19-year-old student presents to her new general practitioner having never had a period. She is otherwise completely well. She is 172 cm tall and weighs 60 kg (body mass index 20 kg/m²). She has never been troubled by her lack of periods, but wonders whether she needs to take contraception.

What further investigations should she have?

What management should you offer?

How would you advise her about her future fertility and her long-term health?

Background

Primary amenorrhoea is the failure to establish normal menstruation.[1,2] Defining the age for investigation is difficult and one could argue that if a young woman is concerned about delay then it should be investigated at that time. In Western society, the majority of girls start menstruating by the age of 13 years and periods usually begin within two years of the development of secondary sexual characteristics. Primary amenorrhoea may be diagnosed when no menstruation has occurred by age 16 years in the presence of normal secondary sexual characteristics. These involve breast development and pubic and axillary hair growth and can be classified using the Tanner system. Oestrogen is required for breast development. Some androgen is required to develop pubic and axillary hair. If, however, there is no secondary sexual development, primary amenorrhoea may be investigated at age 14 years. It is estimated that 0.3% of girls experience primary amenorrhoea.[3]

By far the commonest cause for a delay in the onset of menstruation is *constitutional delay*; this is often familial. However, it can be reassuring to arrange initial investigations to reassure the patient and her family that all appears normal. To achieve puberty, the hypothalamus starts to release gonadotrophin-releasing hormone (GnRH) in a pulsatile fashion. Several factors may contribute to a delay in this development such as low weight, excessive exercise (particularly endurance sport such as running) or stress.[4,5] It may be helpful to address these issues directly.

What further investigations should she have?

The initial categorization of primary amenorrhoea (see Table 7.1) depends on the presence or absence of secondary sexual characteristics and the presence of short stature.

Table 7.1 Causes of primary amenorrhoea
Hypothalamic
Constitutional
Low weight
Stress, exercise
Genetic failure (e.g. Kallman's syndrome)
Chronic illness
Pituitary
Tumour (e.g. prolactinoma)
Gonadal
Gonadal dysgenesis
XX
XO – Turner's syndrome
XY – Androgen insensitivity syndrome
Premature ovarian failure
Polycystic ovaries
Uterine and vaginal
Imperforate hymen
Transverse vaginal septum
Mullerian anomaly (e.g. Rokitansky syndrome)

If the patient also has **short stature**, specialist referral should be considered. In the history, there may be pointers towards hypothalamic damage from trauma or hydrocephalus secondary to infection. Chromosomal abnormality such as Turner's syndrome is associated with short stature and other physical characteristics including webbed neck, wide carrying angle and widely spaced nipples.[6]

If the patient is of **normal height but has no secondary sexual development**, oestrogen is lacking and the cause may be hypothalamic or ovarian. Measuring follicle-stimulating hormone (FSH) will distinguish these two possibilities. A *high FSH level* points towards ovarian failure. Chromosome analysis would then distinguish ovarian failure (or dysgenesis) in an XX or XO female from an XY female, who might have either an enzyme failure, such as androgen insensitivity syndrome (AIS), or gonadal dysgenesis. In an XY phenotypic female, the testicles are usually intra-abdominal or in the groin and should be removed because of the risk of malignant change.

If the *FSH level is normal or low*, a hypothalamic cause is likely. The commonest cause is constitutional delay, as described above. Rarely there is an inheritable defect in the development of the hypothalamus, leading to hypogonadotrophic hypogonadism. This may be associated with defects in the olfactory bulb and anosmia, known as Kallman's syndrome. Fertility can be restored using exogenous pulsatile GnRH.

If the patient has **normal secondary sexual characteristics**, the problem may lie at the hypothalamic/pituitary level, the ovary or with the uterus and vagina. An ultrasound scan will help at this point. It may identify a normal uterus with outflow obstruction. This may be due to an imperforate hymen, which is relatively easy to correct surgically, or a transverse vaginal septum, which tends to be thicker and require more careful surgery.

If the uterus is absent, karyotype is then required. In an *XX female*, the failure of uterine development is called Rokitansky syndrome.[7] Mullerian tract anomalies are associated with renal tract abnormalities. An *XY karyotype* indicates AIS. (Secondary sexual characteristics may develop with AIS due to peripheral conversion of androgen to oestrogen.)

If the uterus is normal, the problem is at the ovarian or hypothalamic/pituitary level. Again, these two possibilities can be distinguished using the FSH level. If the level is high, there is premature ovarian failure (see Case 12: Premature Menopause). Some women with polycystic ovaries (PCO) will present with primary amenorrhoea although secondary amenorrhoea or irregular menstruation would be more common (see Case 8: Irregular Menstruation). In this case, the FSH level would be normal but the luteinizing hormone (LH) level may be raised. An ultrasound scan is the most useful diagnostic tool for PCO.

If the *FSH level is low or normal*, the problem is likely to be hypothalamic or pituitary. Again, constitutional delay would be the most common explanation. Chronic illness and other endocrine abnormalities, such as thyroid disease, may affect the hypothalamus to create amenorrhoea. The prolactin level should be checked and if found to be high a magnetic resonance imaging (MRI) scan of the pituitary fossa should be performed.

What management should you offer?

Initially, a careful history and examination should be performed as in Table 7.2. In the presence of normal growth and normal secondary sexual characteristics, an abdominal ultrasound scan would be the first step (Table 7.3). If this is normal, blood should be taken for analysis of FSH, LH, testosterone and prolactin levels and thyroid function. Karyotyping may then be appropriate. These simple tests are likely to yield sufficient information to categorize the problem roughly and allow appropriate reassurance or referral. It is very important that patients feel that they have had an appropriate explanation for their situation.

Table 7.2 History and examination in primary amenorrhoea
History
Recent weight changes, stresses, exercise habit, eating habits
Chronic illness
Symptoms of thyroid disease
Development of secondary sexual characteristics
Cyclical pain
Galactorrhoea
Family history
Examination
Secondary sexual characteristics
Inspection of external genitalia if possible
Vaginal examination unlikely to be appropriate
Body mass index
Height
Dysmorphic features

Table 7.3 Investigations in primary amenorrhoea
Pelvic ultrasound scan
FSH/LH/testosterone/prolactin level, thyroid function test
Karyotype if raised FSH or abnormal ultrasound (see algorithm)
If prolactin raised, then MRI of pituitary fossa
It may be appropriate to do a pregnancy test

How would you advise her about her future fertility and her long-term health?

Women should be advised that, until proven otherwise, they should consider themselves fertile and use contraception. Questions regarding future fertility should be answered as fully as possible. Not all causes of primary amenorrhoea are associated with low oestrogen levels but, if this is the case, consideration should be given to oestrogen supplementation to protect the skeleton and cardiovascular systems. Oestrogen will have to be combined with a progestogen if the patient has a uterus. This can allow maintenance of bone mass but without gains. There is no evidence regarding bisphosphonates and other non-oestrogen based therapies in this group.

If secondary sexual characteristics are yet to develop, this can be achieved using gradually increasing doses of exogenous oestrogen.

Recent Developments

1 Primary amenorrhoea should be managed initially in primary care but where unusual diagnoses are being considered (e.g. chromosomal abnormalities), referral should probably be made to specialist clinics. The management of these unusual diagnoses is changing rapidly and the views of children, now adults, are increasingly shaping medical care.[8,9]

2 Excessive physical activity can result in exercise related menstrual dysfunction (ERMD), and this can adversely affect the skeleton. The female athlete triad (amenorrhoea, low body mass and osteoporosis) is a well-recognized health issue in female athletes. However, the triad represents the extreme end of the spectrum of exercise related menstrual dysfunction, involving a spectrum of menstrual derangements in females who exercise regularly: amenorrhoea, oligomenorrhoea, anovulation, luteal phase deficiency and delayed menarche.[5] There are also concerns about the increase in risk of infertility and cardiovascular events in later life.

Conclusion

This patient requires a history and examination with the tests described above. If it is found that her amenorrhoea is most likely to be related to excessive exercise, she should be advised to reduce activity as well as take exogenous oestrogen.

Further Reading

1 Edmonds DK. Primary amenorrhea. In: Edmonds DK (ed). *Dewhurst's Textbook of Obstetrics and Gynaecology for Postgraduates*, 7th edn. Oxford: Blackwell Science, 2007; 369–76.

2 Master-Hunter T, Heiman DL. Amenorrhoea: evaluation and treatment. *Am Fam Physician* 2006; **73**: 1374–82.

3 Kiningham RB, Apgar BS, Schwenk TL. Evaluation of amenorrhoea. *Am Fam Physician* 1996; **53**: 1185–94.

4 Mitan LA. Menstrual dysfunction in anorexia nervosa. *J Pediatr Adolesc Gynecol* 2004; **17**: 81–5.

5 Speed C. Exercise-related menstrual dysfunction: implications for menopausal health. *Menopause Int* 2007; **13**: 88–9.

6 Gravholt CH. Clinical practice in Turner syndrome. *Nat Clin Pract Endocrinol Metab* 2005; **1**: 41–52.

7 Guerrier D, Mouchel T, Pasquier L, Pellerin I. The Mayer-Rokitansky-Kuster-Hauser syndrome (congenital absence of uterus and vagina) – phenotypic manifestations and genetic approaches. *J Negat Results Biomed* 2006; **5**: 1.

8 Creighton SM. Adult female outcomes of feminising surgery for ambiguous genitalia. *Pediatr Endocrinol Rev* 2004; **2**: 199–202.

9 Frimberger D, Gearhart JP. Ambiguous genitalia and intersex. *Urol Int* 2005; **75**: 291–7.

08 Irregular Menstruation

Case History

A 25-year-old woman, para 1 (normal vaginal delivery 18 months previously), wants to conceive a second time. She is otherwise fit and well, but since her first child was born her periods now only occur every six to ten weeks. They are heavy but not painful. There is no intermenstrual bleeding. She gained about 12.5 kg during her pregnancy and has never been able to lose it.

What is the most likely explanation for her irregular cycle?

How could the diagnosis be confirmed?

How should this be treated if she did not want to conceive?

What interventions would help to restore her fertility?

What are the long-term implications for her health and fertility?

Background

What is the most likely explanation for her irregular cycle?

The first point is to establish from the history that the pattern of the bleeding is irregular periods and not a chaotic bleeding pattern (Table 8.1). Chaotic bleeding may be due to infection, particularly chlamydia, or to an abnormality within the uterus such as a polyp or endometrial carcinoma. Abnormalities on the cervix, such as an ectropion or a carcinoma, may also present with irregular bleeding but this would often be associated with post-coital bleeding as well.

The commonest cause of irregular menstruation is polycystic ovaries (PCO), accounting for 80% of cases. Other causes include premature menopause and anovulation, perhaps due to hormonal contraception. With polycystic ovary syndrome (PCOS) the fundamental lesion appears to be increased insulin resistance, perhaps due to an inherited defect in the insulin receptor. Hormone production within the ovary is abnormal. There is also a reduction in the level of sex hormone binding globulin which leads to an increase in free testosterone. Ovulation fails to occur and without the progesterone produced by the corpus luteum, the menstrual cycle tends to be prolonged and irregular.[1]

Table 8.1 Features in the history and examination

History

    Nature of cycle, intermenstrual/post-coital bleeding, menorrhagia

    Previous pattern of bleeding

    Recent weight changes/stresses

    Fertility aspirations

    Breast-feeding

    Other symptoms:

        Acne, hirsutism, hot flushes, vaginal discharge, pain

    Smear history

    Contraceptive history

    Sexual history

    Family history

Examination

    Body mass index

    Blood pressure

    Signs of virilization or hyperpigmentation

    Degree of hirsutism (Feriman–Gallwey score)

    Pelvic mass or tenderness

How could the diagnosis be confirmed?

To make the diagnosis of PCOS, two out of the following three criteria should be met: ultrasound evidence of PCO on transvaginal ultrasound scan; clinical or biochemical evidence of hyperandrogenism; and evidence of anovulation (see Table 8.2). Blood tests may show evidence of hyperandrogenism. Testosterone levels of 3–5 nmol/l would not be unusual in PCOS, but levels above this raise the possibility of an androgen-secreting tumour. Androstenedione is an androgen which arises primarily from the ovary and may be raised in PCOS.

Approximately 20% of the female population have ultrasound evidence of PCO (i.e. purely morphological changes). About 10% have PCOS (i.e. clinical abnormalities associated with PCO).[2] This is so common as to be almost normal and there are those who consider it to be a physiological variant, perhaps allowing populations to survive during times of starvation.[3]

Table 8.2 Diagnostic criteria for polycystic ovary syndrome (PCOS)

For diagnosis of PCOS, two of the three following criteria should be met:

- Ultrasound evidence of PCO
- (>12 follicles, 2–9 mm diameter or ovarian volume >10 cm³)
- Clinical or biochemical evidence of hyperandrogenism
- Menstrual irregularity or anovulation

How should this be treated if she did not want to conceive?

Weight reduction is central to the management of PCOS. High body mass index (BMI) increases insulin resistance and exacerbates symptoms.[4] A 5%–10% reduction in weight may be sufficient to allow menstruation to return. Some advocate a low-carbohydrate diet to aid weight reduction in PCOS. Dieticians can be very helpful in helping the patient to define a healthy diet and to identify psychological patterns which may block weight reduction.

The features of PCOS can be treated on a purely symptomatic basis. Hirsutism can be addressed using systemic or local treatments; waxing or laser treatment may be sufficient. Eflornithine hydrochloride cream is a useful adjuvant to reduce hair growth. Spironolactone can be used systemically. It is well tolerated and has some anti-androgenic activity. Powerful anti-androgens such as finasteride may be justified, but effective contraception must be used to avoid feminization of a male fetus. Acne may be treated with local or systemic antibiotic and steroid protocols.[5]

To treat irregular bleeding as well as the androgenic effects, the combined contraceptive pill may be used. One often chosen contains the anti-androgen progestogen cyproterone acetate, but other pills may be just as effective. It should not normally be used for longer than 6–12 months because of its adverse effect on lipid profiles and the higher thrombotic risk compared to other contraceptive pills.

What interventions would help to restore her fertility?

Patients should be advised that their BMI should be as near normal as possible before embarking on fertility treatment. Being overweight during pregnancy increases the risks of pregnancy for both mother and baby (see Case 20: Optimizing Assisted Conception). Miscarriage and infertility are more common in overweight women. Ovulation induction is less likely to be successful and much harder to monitor in obese women. Losing weight alone may be all that is required to re-establish ovulation. Ideally, the BMI should be less than 30 kg/m^2 before the initiation of fertility treatment.[6]

Clomifene citrate can be used to induce ovulation. Most women have few side effects on this regime, although if double vision occurs the drug should be stopped. Clomifene is taken from day 2 to day 6 of the cycle and follicular monitoring is essential in the first cycle to ensure that the dose is correct. Too small a dose will not induce ovulation; too high may generate more than two follicles with the resulting risk of high-order multiple pregnancy. It may be necessary to induce a bleed using a progestogen before starting the clomifene. If clomifene is unsuccessful, other methods of ovulation induction can be explored (see Cases 19: Assisted Conception Methods and 20: Optimizing Assisted Conception).

What are the long-term implications for her health and fertility?

In the longer term, women with PCOS should be aware of two potential health risks. Firstly, the unopposed oestrogen associated with anovulatory cycles may result in prolonged stimulation of the endometrium. This may cause hyperplasia or even carcinoma within the endometrium even in relatively young women under 40 years of age. A change in menstrual pattern, particularly the development of a chaotic bleeding pattern, should prompt further investigation to sample the endometrium. Women with PCOS should be aware that it is important to have at least three or four periods a year to shed the endometrium. These may happen spontaneously or can be induced using the combined oral contraceptive pill or periodic progestogen.

Secondly, women with PCOS are at increased risk of diabetes and should be screened appropriately as they get older. This risk is increased in overweight women. Women with PCOS should be screened for gestational diabetes during pregnancy.[7]

Recent Developments

Metformin is becoming widely used in the treatment of PCOS. It acts to reduce insulin levels by sensitizing peripheral tissues to the action of insulin. It is taken in a dose of 2 g daily but side effects may be limiting. Most commonly, side effects are gastrointestinal: diarrhoea, bloating, nausea, etc. These can be reduced by introducing the dose slowly. The use of metformin to induce ovulation has attracted attention but the results are contradictory[8,9] (see Case 20: Optimizing Assisted Conception). There is, however, only limited evidence that it is effective in treating any other symptoms of PCOS, including obesity.[10]

Conclusion

PCOS cannot be cured, but women should be aware of its implications for their long-term health and fertility and be informed about available options for managing their own condition. The obesity epidemic is highlighting the health and socio-economic consequences of being overweight. It is therefore essential to emphasize the need for weight loss and maintenance of a normal BMI.

Further Reading

1 Balen A. The current understanding of polycystic ovary syndrome. *The Obstetrician and Gynaecologist* 2004; **6**: 66–74.

2 Michelmore KF, Balen AH, Dunger DB, Vessey MP. Polycystic ovaries and associated clinical and biochemical features in young women. *Clin Endocrinol* 1999; **51**: 779–86.

3 Gleicher N, Barad D. An evolutionary concept of polycystic ovarian disease: does evolution favour reproductive success over survival? *Reprod Biomed Online* 2006; **12**: 587–9.

4 Barber TM, McCarthy MI, Wass JA, Franks S. Obesity and polycystic ovary syndrome. *Clin Endocrinol* 2006; **65**: 137–45.

5 Moghetti P, Toscano V. Treatment of hirsutism and acne in hyperandrogenism. *Best Pract Res Clin Endocrinol Metab* 2006; **20**: 221–34.

6 Homburg R. Pregnancy complications in PCOS. *Best Pract Res Clin Endocrinol Metab* 2006; **20**: 281–92.

7 Royal College of Obstetricians and Gynaecologists (RCOG). *Long-Term Consequences of Polycystic Ovary Syndrome*. Green-top Guideline No. 33. London: RCOG Press, 2003.

8   Lord JM, Flight IHK, Norman RJ. Insulin sensitising drugs for polycystic ovary syndrome. *The Cochrane Library*, Issue 4. Chichester: John Wiley & Sons, 2006.

9   Legro RS, Barnhart HX, Schlaff WD, Carr BR, Diamond MP, Carson SA, Steinkampf MP, Coutifaris C, McGovern PG, Cataldo NA, Gosman GG, Nestler JE, Giudice LC, Leppert PC, Myers ER; Cooperative Multicenter Reproductive Medicine Network. Clomiphene, metformin, or both for infertility in the polycystic ovary syndrome. *N Engl J Med* 2007; **356**: 551–66.

10 Lord J, Wilkin T. Metformin in polycystic ovary syndrome. *Curr Opin Obstet Gynecol* 2004; **16**: 481–6.

09 Premenstrual Syndrome

Case History

Dr Oat is a 36-year-old museum curator with two children. She finds that she is 'like Jekyll and Hyde': two weeks of her cycle she is a warm, loving mother and wife, and calm, facilitating work colleague, but for the ten days before her period she knows she screams at the children, hates her staff and feels very miserable and 'out of control'. She cannot bear going on like this.

How should you assess her?

What are the treatment options?

Background

Many women notice changes in their emotional and physical feelings during the menstrual cycle. These disturbances are very variable. Different women have different symptoms and these may vary from month to month in both type and severity. There are no biochemical or other physical markers for the condition and premenstrual syndrome (PMS) may represent several heterogeneous syndromes.[1] O'Brien gives the definition '...a disorder of non-specific somatic, psychological or behavioural symptoms recurring in the premenstrual phase of the menstrual cycle. Symptoms must resolve completely by the end of menstruation leaving a symptom-free week' (see Table 9.1). 'The symptoms should be of sufficient severity to produce social, family or occupational disruption. Symptoms must have occurred in at least four of the six previous menstrual cycles'.[2] The symptoms vary but the most common ones include low mood, irritability, feeling out of control, anxiety, tension, clumsiness, poor memory, food craving, sleep disturbance, bloating, breast tenderness, abdominal pain, backache, weight gain and fatigue.

How should you assess her?

Essential questions to ask are:

- How long has this been going on?
- What contraception is she using?
- What is her past psychiatric history?

Women should be asked to complete menstrual charts, recording their moods and other symptoms for at least two cycles. Three patterns may emerge:

1 True PMS
2 The menstrual pattern orchestrating underlying psychological problems that are there all the time (e.g. anxiety/depression)
3 Psychological problems unrelated to the menstrual cycle but falsely attributed to it

Table 9.1 DSM-IV* criteria for premenstrual dysphoric disorder

DSM-IV criteria for premenstrual dysphoric disorder

- In most menstrual cycles during the past year, five (or more) of the following symptoms were present for most of the time during the last week of the luteal phase, began to remit during menses and were absent in the week post-menses:
    - low mood, hopelessness, self-deprecating thoughts
    - anxiety, tension, edginess
    - lability of mood
    - anger, irritability, loss of interest
    - poor concentration
    - lethargy, fatigue
    - overeating or cravings
    - hypersomnia or insomnia
    - feeling overwhelmed, out of control
    - physical symptoms (e.g. breast tenderness, bloating, headaches, joint aches, weight gain)
- The syndrome markedly disturbs work or school and relationships
- Disturbance is not an exacerbation of another disorder
- Criteria above must be confirmed by prospective daily symptom ratings for at least two consecutive months

*DSM-IV: Diagnostic and Statistical Manual of Mental Disorders, 4th Edition

What are the treatment options?

A variety of treatment options are available (see Table 9.2).

Listening and explaining

The first and most important approach is actually to listen to the woman and take her complaint seriously. Often they have asked other doctors for help in the past without success. Understanding where the woman is coming from and what she may or may not perceive about herself and her hormones may be the most therapeutic option. The one consistent factor in the few randomized controlled trials on any of the PMS treatments is the very high placebo response (about 60% improvement), so try harmless treatments first! Regular exercise is a mood improver and helps general fitness. Women should do 20 minutes exercise three times a week, which will also improve cardiovascular fitness and bone strength. Some women find a 'no sugar' diet very helpful, and particularly no chocolate, but there has not been a randomized controlled trial on this.

Supplements

Oil of evening primrose is good for relieving breast tenderness.[3] Pyridoxine (vitamin B6) 50 mg twice daily helps in mild PMS,[4] but can cause a neuropathy in excessive doses. Vitex agnus castus fruit extract helps PMS.[5] In the United Kingdom, women regard St John's wort as a herbal remedy; it is really a selective serotonin reuptake inhibitor (SSRI; see below), but it does work probably because of this property.

Hormonal manipulation

Oestrogen has antidopaminergic properties and progesterone modulates gamma-aminobutyric acid, the neurotransmitter involved in emotional control. Since true PMS is in some way caused by the fluctuation of hormones in the second half of the menstrual cycle, wiping out the cycle by various means may be effective. If this is not effective, the woman does not have PMS. If the woman needs contraception, continuous oral contraception should help, as does (in some) the levonorgestrel-releasing intrauterine device, although it may make some women worse. Oestrogen 100 μg patches are effective,[6] and in extreme, unresponsive cases, treatment may resort to an artificial menopause with gonadotrophin-releasing hormone agonists, with add-back oestrogen therapy. The role of progesterone is uncertain and a systematic review, which found only two trials suitable for inclusion, concluded that 'We could not say that progesterone helped women with PMS, nor that it was ineffective'.[7] The menopause ends PMS.

Selective serotonin reuptake inhibitors (SSRIs)

There is evidence of a serotonergic mechanism in the blunted prolactin response to fenfluramine, which is supported by the finding that the serotonin reuptake inhibiting antidepressants (e.g. fluoxetine, paroxetine, sertraline, citalopram) are effective in treating PMS.[8,9] What is odd is that they seem to work administered either continuously or intermittently in the second half of the cycle only. This effect has been postulated to arise from the cyclical nature of PMS and may reflect SSRI action at a different receptor site from that in affective disorders. Some women find it more acceptable to take antidepressants intermittently, rather than feeling 'addicted' to them.

Table 9.2 Treatment for PMS
Treatment for PMS
● Nutritional supplements: evening primrose oil, pyridoxine, magnesium, zinc, vitex agnus castus fruit, special low-sugar no-chocolate diets
● Psychosocial: lifestyle adjustment, relaxation training, cognitive behavioural therapy
● Antidepressants: SSRIs
● Hormones: oestrogen, progesterone, progestogens
● Gonadotrophin-releasing hormone agonists

Cognitive behavioural therapy

One could argue that cognitive behavioural therapy is an odd way of approaching an hormonally induced change of mood, yet it improves PMS.[10] It does not change the PMS, but changes the way a woman copes with and looks at her life, identifying solvable problems, and not getting upset by unsolvable ones.

Recent Developments

1   The results of twin and family studies suggest that PMS is a heritable disorder. Genotypic differences are likely to mediate a differential behavioural response to gonadal steroids. An association has been found between allelic variants in the oestrogen receptor alpha gene and PMS.[11]

2   Health professionals must be prepared to encounter patients with PMS who are considering pregnancy. The American College of Obstetricians and Gynecologists (ACOG) treatment guidelines for the management of premenstrual symptoms recommend SSRIs as the preferred method for treating PMS.[12] Overall, the data regarding the safety of SSRIs during pregnancy are limited and inconclusive. Therefore, patients should be advised that the reproductive safety of these medications has not been well established or adequately studied to draw definitive conclusions, and the issue remains controversial.

Conclusion

PMS is long-term condition that will only stop after the menopause and thus this patient can expect about another 15 years of symptoms. The patient decides to try cognitive behavioural therapy as this will also help with dealing with life at home or at work.

Further Reading

1   Blake F. Psychological aspects of gynaecology. In: Rees M, Hope S (eds). *Specialist Training in Gynaecology*. Edinburgh: Elsevier Mosby, 2005; 200–15.

2 O'Brien PMS. The premenstrual syndrome. *Br J Family Plann* 1990; **15**(Suppl): 13–18.

3 Budeiri DJ, Li Wan Po A, Dornan JC. Is evening primrose oil of value in the treatment of the premenstrual syndrome? *Control Clin Trials* 1996; **17**: 60–8.

4 Wyatt KM, Dimmock PW, Jones PW, O'Brien PMS. Efficacy of vitamin B-6 in the treatment of premenstrual syndrome: systematic review. *BMJ* 1999; **318**: 1375–81.

5 Schellenberg R. Treatment for the premenstrual syndrome with agnus castus fruit extract: prospective, randomised, placebo controlled study. *BMJ* 2001; **322**: 134–7.

6 Smith RN, Studd JWW, Zamblera D, Holland EFN. A randomised comparison over 8 months of 100 micrograms and 200 micrograms twice weekly doses of transdermal oestradiol in the treatment of severe premenstrual syndrome. *Br J Obstet Gynaecol* 1995; **102**: 475–84.

7 Ford O, Lethaby A, Mol B, Roberts H. Progesterone for premenstrual syndrome. *Cochrane Database Syst Rev* 2006; CD003415.

8 Wyatt KM, Dimmock PW, O'Brien PM. Selective serotonin reuptake inhibitors for premenstrual syndrome. *Cochrane Database Syst Rev* 2002; CD001396.

9 Landen M, Nissbrandt H, Allgulander C, Sorvik K, Ysander C, Eriksson E. Placebo-controlled trial comparing intermittent and continuous paroxetine in premenstrual dysphoric disorder. *Neuropsychopharmacology* 2007; **32**: 153–61.

10 Blake F, Salkovskis P, Gath D, Day A, Garrod A. Cognitive therapy for premenstrual syndrome: a controlled trial. *J Psychosom Res* 1998; **45**: 307–18.

11 Huo L, Straub RE, Schmidt PJ, Shi K, Vakkalanka R, Weinberger DR, Rubinow DR. Risk for Premenstrual Dysphoric Disorder Is Associated with Genetic Variation in ESR1, the Estrogen Receptor Alpha Gene. *Biol Psychiatry* 2007; [Epub ahead of print].

12 American College of Obstetricians and Gynecologists. Premenstrual syndrome. ACOG practice bulletin no. 15, American College of Obstetricians and Gynecologists, Washington, DC. 2000. Available at National Guidelines Clearinghouse: www.guideline.gov/summary/summary.aspx?ss=15&doc_id=3965&nbr=3103 (accessed 16 10 07)

PROBLEM

10 Alternative and Complementary Therapies for Menorrhagia and Dysmenorrhoea

Case History

A 25-year-old woman attends complaining of heavy, painful periods. She is not keen to use conventional medication and asks about alternative and complementary therapies.

What are the available preparations?

What is the evidence of efficacy?

What is the safety profile of these preparations?

Background

The use of alternative and complementary therapies (ACTs) for a range of medical conditions is becoming increasingly popular. The National Omnibus Survey in the United Kingdom found that an estimated 10% of the population had used any ACT from a practitioner in the previous year, and more than half of these had not informed their general practitioner.[1]

Menstrual problems are very common in young women and for a number of reasons these women may be reluctant to use prescribed medicines to alleviate symptoms. Many women believe that ACTs are 'safer' but there are limited published data to confirm safety or, indeed, efficacy.[2] Most ACTs (Table 10.1) have been used for the relief of symptoms of primary and secondary dysmenorrhoea.

Table 10.1 Alternative and complementary therapies used for menstrual problems		
Herbal preparations	**Vitamins and minerals**	**Others**
Sweet fennel	Calcium and magnesium	Acupuncture
Vitex agnus castus	Vitamin B1	Aromatherapy
Rose tea	Vitamin E	
Pycnogenol		
Toki-shakuyaku-san		
Traditional Chinese medicine		

Herbal preparations

Herbal and dietary therapies are often used to treat primary and secondary dysmenorrhoea. In the United States (US), herbs and other phytomedicinal products have been legally classified as dietary supplements since 1994.[2]

Sweet fennel has been compared with mefenamic acid for the treatment of primary dysmenorrhoea. In one study, efficacy was assessed using a self-scoring system over three cycles.[3] Mefenamic acid had a more potent effect than fennel on the second and third menstrual days; however, the difference on the other days was not significant. Fennel was therefore concluded to be a safe and effective remedy, although may need to be used in higher dosages to increase potency.

Vitex agnus castus (VAC) is a deciduous shrub, native to Mediterranean Europe and Central Asia. VAC fruit extract has been used for the treatment of a range of gynaecological conditions and the German Commission E has approved its use for irregularities of the menstrual cycle, premenstrual disturbances and mastodynia.[4] Available evidence suggests that adverse effects are mild and reversible, with few drug interactions.[4]

Rose tea ingestion has been used for the treatment of primary dysmenorrhoea. A study in Taiwan reported a reduction in menstrual pain, distress and anxiety and greater psychophysiologic well-being at one, three and six months after intervention in adolescents randomized to drinking rose tea compared to controls.[5]

Pycnogenol (PYC), a standardized extract of French maritime pine bark, has been shown to have a number of beneficial pharmacological properties and has been used in a range of medical conditions. It has been shown to reduce premenstrual symptoms, including abdominal cramps.[6] PYC is primarily composed of procyanidins and phenolic acids, and its mechanism of action in this case is likely to be due to the spasmolytic action of phenolic acids.

Toki-shakuyaku-san is a traditional Japanese herbal combination which has been used as a remedy for amenorrhoea, luteal phase dysfunction and dysmenorrhoea.[2] Studies of this herbal combination are limited.

Traditional Chinese medicine uses a combination of up to 20 different herbs, adjusted according to each individual case. Limited studies have shown some efficacy in the treatment of dysmenorrhoea and it is postulated that these particular herbal combinations act by decreasing prostaglandin levels, modulating nitric oxide, increasing plasma β-endorphin levels, blocking calcium channels and improving the microcirculation.[7]

Vitamins and minerals

Calcium and magnesium. There is evidence to suggest that fluctuating levels of ovarian hormones influence calcium, magnesium and vitamin D metabolism.[8] Studies have shown promising results using magnesium supplementation to treat women with primary dysmenorrhoea[9,10] but patient numbers are small. One study measured prostaglandin F2α (PGF2α) levels in menstrual blood and found a correlation between magnesium therapy, declining PGF2α levels and improved symptoms of primary dysmenorrhoea over a six-month period.[11] This effect, along with the muscle relaxant and vasodilatory action of magnesium, may in part explain its therapeutic effect. Calcium has largely been studied for its beneficial effect on premenstrual symptoms. A study in the US randomly assigned 497 healthy women between the ages of 18 and 45 years to receive either calcium carbonate 1200 mg daily or placebo for three menstrual cycles.[12] At the end of the third cycle, there was a 48% reduction in all four symptom scores, including negative affect, water retention, food cravings and pain.

Vitamin B1 plays an important role in metabolism, and deficiency may result in a number of symptoms including fatigue, muscle cramps and reduced pain tolerance.[2] One study using therapeutic thiamine reports benefit for the symptoms of moderate to severe spasmodic primary dysmenorrhoea.[13] This study randomized 556 girls, aged 12–21 years, to receive either 100 mg thiamine orally or placebo for 90 days. The combined final results of both the 'active treatment first' group and the 'placebo first' group after 90 days of treatment were 87% completely cured, 8% relieved (pain almost nil to reduced) and 5% showed no effect whatsoever.

Vitamin E. It has been suggested that Vitamin E has analgesic and anti-inflammatory properties[2] and may therefore be useful for the treatment of dysmenorrhoea. Studies, however, are needed to support this claim.

Dietary interventions

Omega-3 fatty acids. Levels of polyunsaturated fatty acids (PUFAs) are associated with menstrual pain, with higher levels of omega-3 fatty acids associated with a reduction in menstrual symptoms.[2] PUFAs are metabolized into specific prostaglandins associated with dysmenorrhoea and the ratio of omega-3 to omega-6 fatty acids, obtained by dietary means, may be of significance.

Others

Acupuncture is becoming increasingly popular for the treatment of a wide range of medical conditions in the Western world. One study randomized 61 women with moderately severe primary dysmenorrhoea to acupressure or no treatment. Acupressure was applied using the 'Relief Brief', a garment with a fixed number of lower abdominal and lower back latex foam acupads that provide pressure to dysmenorrhoea-relieving Chinese acupressure points.[14] Almost all (90%) of the women wearing the Relief Brief experienced at least a 25% reduction in menstrual pain severity, compared to only 8% of the control group; median pain medication use dropped from six to two pills per day for the acupressure group but remained at six pills per day for the controls at the end of two menstrual cycles.

Aromatherapy has also been applied for the relief of a number of menstrual symptoms, including dysmenorrhoea. One study randomized 67 women with dysmenorrhoea to receive either aromatherapy using lavender, clary sage and rose in almond oil (the treatment group), aromatherapy with almond oil alone (the placebo group) or no treatment (the control group).[15] Menstrual cramps were significantly reduced on both the first and second days of the cycle in the treatment group compared to the two other groups.

Recent Developments

The use of ACTs in Europe and North America is increasing significantly. Users are educated and self-empowered and rely on information sources beyond mainstream medical practitioners. Not surprisingly, media coverage, much of dubious quality, has increased to meet demand for information. A survey of media information suggests that there were significant errors of omission in describing clinical trial quality and a serious under-reporting of risks of herbal remedies.[16] Thus users of ACTs are not being provided with information sufficient to make informed choices about treatment alternatives.

Conclusion

Clearly, the use of alternative and complementary therapies for the relief of menstrual symptoms is expanding and increasing in popularity among women who choose to avoid conventional medicines. However, more studies are needed to prove not only efficacy but also safety before their use can be confidently recommended. Interactions with hormonal contraception reducing contraceptive efficacy have also to be discussed.

Further Reading

1　Thomas K, Coleman P. Use of complementary or alternative medicine in a general population in Great Britain. Results from the National Omnibus Survey. *J Public Health (Oxf)* 2004; **26**: 152–7.

2　Rees M, Hope S, Ravnikar V (eds). *The Abnormal Menstrual Cycle*. Abingdon: Taylor and Francis, 2005.

3　Jahromi BN, Tartifizadeh A, Khabnadideh S. Comparison of fennel and mefenamic acid for the treatment of primary dysmenorrhoea. *Int J Gynaecol Obstet* 2003; **80**: 153–7.

4　Daniele C, Coon JT, Pittler MH, Ernst E. Vitex agnus castus: a systematic review of adverse events. *Drug Saf* 2005; **28**: 319–32.

5　Tseng YF, Chen CH, Yang YH. Rose tea for relief of primary dysmenorrhoea in adolescents: a randomized controlled trial in Taiwan. *J Midwifery Womens Health* 2005; **50**: 51–7.

6　Rohdewald P. A review of the French maritime pine bark extract (Pycnogenol), a herbal medication with a diverse clinical pharmacology. *Int J Clin Pharmacol Ther* 2002; **40**: 158–68.

7　Jia W, Wang X, Xu D, Zhao A, Zhang Y. Common traditional Chinese medicinal herbs for dysmenorrhoea. *Phytother Res* 2006; **20**: 819–24.

8　Thys-Jacobs S. Micronutrients and the premenstrual syndrome: the case for calcium. *J Am Coll Nutr* 2000; **19**: 220–7.

9　Benassi L, Barletta FP, Baroncini L, Bertani D, Filippini F, Beski L, Nani A, Tesauri P, Tridenti G. Effectiveness of magnesium pidolate in the prophylactic treatment of primary dysmenorrhea. *Clin Exp Obstet Gynecol* 1992; **19**: 176–9.

10　Proctor ML, Murphy PA. Herbal and dietary therapies for primary and secondary dysmenorrhoea. *Cochrane Database Syst Rev* 2001; CD002124.

11　Seifert B, Wagler P, Dartsch S, Schmidt U, Nieder J. Magnesium – a new therapeutic alternative in primary dysmenorrhea. *Zentralbl Gynakol* 1989; **111**: 755–60.

12 Thys-Jacobs S, Starkey P, Bernstein D, Tian J. Calcium carbonate and the premenstrual syndrome: effects on premenstrual and menstrual symptoms. Premenstrual Syndrome Study Group. *Am J Obstet Gynecol* 1998; **179**: 444–52.

13 Gokhale LB. Curative treatment of primary (spasmodic) dysmenorrhoea. *Indian J Med Res* 1996; **103**: 227–31.

14 Taylor D, Miaskowski C, Kohn J. A randomized clinical trial of the effectiveness of an acupressure device (Relief Brief) for managing symptoms of dysmenorrhea. *J Altern Complement Med* 2002; **8**: 357–70.

15 Han SH, Hur MH, Buckle J, Choi J, Lee MS. Effect of aromatherapy on symptoms of dysmenorrhea in college students: a randomized placebo-controlled clinical trial. *J Altern Complement Med* 2006; **12**: 535–41.

16 Bubela T, Koper M, Boon H, Caulfield T. Media portrayal of herbal remedies versus pharmaceutical clinical trials: impacts on decision. *Med Law* 2007; **26**: 363–73.

Menopause

PROBLEM

11 Peri-menopausal Menstrual Symptoms

Case History

A 46-year-old woman complains of irregular heavy periods every four to six weeks over the past year and is flushing. She is using condoms for contraception and her family is complete.

What are the issues?

How should she be investigated?

What are the treatments?

Background

What are the issues?

Menopausal symptoms often start before menstruation stops and this patient would benefit from trying hormone replacement therapy (HRT). However, before then it is important to ascertain her contraceptive needs and to exclude pelvic pathology and to ensure that she is not anaemic.

How should she be investigated?

Evaluation begins with a detailed history focusing on menstrual patterns, subjective heaviness of loss (such as passage of clots) and vasomotor symptoms. An abdominal and pelvic examination is recommended. Cervical cytology should be up-to-date in accordance with local screening programmes. A full blood count is needed to determine the degree of anaemia.[1] In a woman of her age there is no need to check follicle-stimulating hormone (FSH) levels. They fluctuate in the peri-menopause, will not predict when periods will stop and are not a guide to fertility status, as ovulation can occur in the presence of elevated FSH levels. However, it would be prudent to check thyroid function as thyroid disease is very common in women.[2] Transvaginal ultrasound scanning (TVS) should then be used as a triage for further diagnostic evaluation (Figure 11.1). It will diagnose endometrial pathologies, including polyps and submucous fibroids, as well as other pelvic pathologies such as ovarian cysts. While endometrial thickness is an indicator of pathology in post-menopausal women, there are no such clear guidelines in peri-menopausal women. The United Kingdom 'Royal College of Obstetricians and Gynaecologists Guideline Development Group' reviewed a number of studies involving pre-menopausal women and concluded that 10–12 mm represented a reasonable cut-off when using TVS as a method prior to more invasive procedures of endometrial assessment.[3] Ideally, TVS should be performed after menstruation in the follicular phase of the menstrual cycle. Ultrasound can sometimes miss small polyps, particularly when

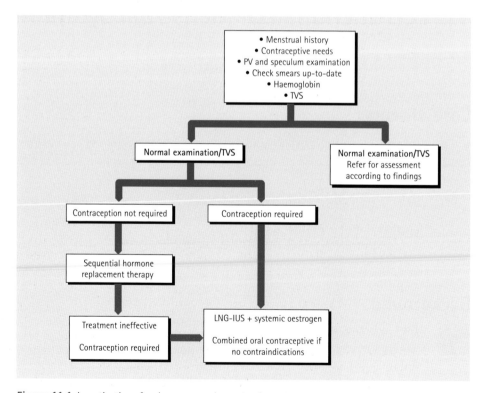

Figure 11.1 Investigation of peri-menopausal menstrual symptoms.

performed in the late secretory phase when the endometrium is thicker. Endometrial sampling should be considered in this woman to obtain a histological diagnosis to exclude malignant and pre-malignant disease. This is usually undertaken without anaesthetic using a Pipelle sampler. However, if endometrial pathology such as an endometrial polyp is suspected, direct visualization with hysteroscopy is preferred and the lesion can then be removed. Of course if gross pelvic pathology such as large fibroids is found, she will need to be referred for consideration for surgery.

What are the treatments?

Medical treatments are the first line if no gross pelvic pathology requiring surgery is found. She could try non-hormonal treatments such as mefenamic acid and tranexamic acid to reduce her blood loss; however, this would not address either her menopausal symptoms or her contraceptive needs. If she wishes to try HRT she would need to try a sequential regimen since she is peri-menopausal. While studies that have measured withdrawal bleeds on sequential therapy have found them to be no heavier than normal menstruations, there is no good evidence that therapy will reduce excessive menstrual bleeding.[4] Also, HRT will not provide contraception.

Depo-Provera (intramuscular medroxyprogesterone acetate), despite being licensed as a contraceptive, is often used to treat menorrhagia as it can induce amenorrhoea, especially after repeated injections. However, no randomized controlled trials have addressed its use in menorrhagia at any age, there would be concerns about osteoporosis in this age group and there are no data about concomitant systemic oestrogen.[5] There are no data about the use of the progestogen-only pill in menorrhagia and, furthermore, none about its use in women taking systemic oestrogen.[6]

Combined oral contraceptives (COCs) are commonly used in younger women to provide contraception, regulate their menstrual cycles and reduce menstrual blood loss. However, as women move into the peri-menopause they are probably under-used.[7] More women in this age group will have contraindications to the COC but non-smokers with no additional cardiovascular risk factors can safely use it until the age of 50 years. However, data about use for peri-menopausal menstrual problems are scant. If she is found to be anaemic she will require iron supplements.

Recent Developments

Treatment has been revolutionized with the introduction of the levonorgestrel-releasing intrauterine system (LNG-IUS), or Mirena®. It is licensed for contraception and menorrhagia and provides the progestogen component for HRT regimens. She could then take systemic oestrogen using the route of her choice: oral or transdermal. A systematic review on the LNG-IUS indicates it results in a significant reduction in menstrual blood loss from baseline in heavy menstrual bleeding.[8] It is more effective and acceptable to women than 21 days of oral norethisterone taken cyclically but there are still only a few randomized controlled trials. The device is not as effective as endometrial ablation at reducing menstrual blood loss but this does not appear to affect women's satisfaction. It is more cost-effective than hysterectomy both in the short term (one year) and longer term (five years).[9] She will need to be advised that she may have irregular, unpredictable bleeding during the first six months after insertion of the LNG-IUS. Of note, a study based on data gathered from a large post-marketing study on LNG-IUS users ($n = 17\,360$) in Finland found that the LNG-IUS was not associated with an increased risk of breast cancer.[10]

Conclusion

Peri-menopausal menstrual problems are common. This woman has three issues: menstrual problems, menopausal symptoms and a need for effective contraception. The management plan is to address all three as well as excluding pathology.

Further Reading

1 CKS. Clinical topic. Menorrhagia (heavy menstrual bleeding). www.cks.library.nhs.uk/menorrhagia (accessed 20 09 07)

2 Pearce E. Thyroid dysfunction in perimenopausal and postmenopausal women. *Menopause Int* 2007; **13**: 8–13.

3 Royal College of Obstetricians and Gynaecologists (RCOG). *The Management of Menorrhagia in Secondary Care*. Evidence-Based Clinical Guideline No. 5. London: RCOG, 1999.

4 Rees MC, Barlow DH. Quantitation of hormone replacement induced withdrawal bleeds. *Br J Obstet Gynaecol* 1991; **98**: 106–7.

5 Rees M, Purdie DW (eds). *Managment of the Menopause: The Handbook*. London: Royal Society of Medicine Press, 2006.

6 Duckitt K. Medical management of perimenopausal menorrhagia: an evidence-based approach. *Menopause Int* 2007; **13**: 14–18.

7 Faculty of Family Planning and Reproductive Health Care. UK Medical Eligibility Criteria for Contraceptive Use (UKMEC 2005/2006). www.ffprhc.org.uk (accessed 20 09 07)

8 Lethaby AE, Cooke I, Rees M. Progesterone or progestogen-releasing intrauterine systems for heavy menstrual bleeding. *Cochrane Database Syst Rev* 2005; CD002126.

9 Hurskainen R, Teperi J, Rissanen P, Aalto AM, Grenman S, Kivela A, Kujansuu E, Vuorma S, Yliskoski M, Paavonen J. Clinical outcomes and costs with the levonorgestrel-releasing intrauterine system or hysterectomy for treatment of menorrhagia: randomized trial 5-year follow-up. *JAMA* 2004; **291**: 1456–63.

10 Backman T, Rauramo I, Jaakkola K, Inki P, Vaahtera K, Launonen A, Koskenvuo M. Use of the levonorgestrel-releasing intrauterine system and breast cancer. *Obstet Gynecol* 2005; **106**: 813–17.

12 Premature Menopause

Case History

A 29-year-old woman presents with irregular periods and hot flushes for the past four months. She has two normally developed boys and is using a copper-bearing intrauterine device for contraception. Her mother became menopausal at the age of 35 years.

What tests should you do?

What are the long-term health implications?

What treatment should you recommend?

What are the fertility/contraception issues?

Background

Premature ovarian failure (POF) is common.[1,2] It is estimated to affect 1% of women younger than 40 years and 0.1% of those under 30 years. It can present as primary or secondary amenorrhoea. In the great majority of cases, no cause can be found. Women with POF frequently have autoimmune disorders, particularly hypothyroidism (25%), Addison's disease (3%) and diabetes mellitus (2.5%). Other coexisting conditions may include Crohn's disease, vitiligo, pernicious anaemia, systemic lupus erythematosus or rheumatoid arthritis. While follicle-stimulating hormone (FSH) receptor gene polymorphisms, inhibin B mutations and enzyme deficiencies can cause POF, presentation is at a much younger age. A critical region on the X-chromosome (POF1), ranging from Xq13 to Xq26, which relates to normal ovarian function has been identified, as has a second gene of paternal origin (POF2), which is located at Xq13.3–q21.1. Idiopathic POF can be familial or sporadic, and the familial pattern of inheritance is compatible with X-linked inheritance with incomplete penetrance or an autosomal dominant mode of inheritance. Familial POF has been linked with fragile X permutations. Although women with POF are generally considered to be infertile, spontaneous ovarian activity may occur with the resulting implications of fertility and pregnancy.

What tests should you do?

A diagnosis of POF must be made with two FSH measurements preferably during menstruation or two weeks apart if periods are very infrequent.[2] Other endocrine disease (such as thyroid dysfunction) that can also cause hot flushes and menstrual irregularity should be excluded (Table 12.1). Coexisting disease must be detected, particularly

Table 12.1	Investigation of premature menopause

- Estimates of levels of follicle-stimulating hormone in serum (×2)
- Thyroid function tests
- Autoimmune screen for polyendocrinopathy
- Chromosome analysis, especially in women younger than 30 years
- Estimates of bone mineral density through dual-energy X-ray absorptiometry (optional)
- Adrenocorticotrophic hormone stimulation test if Addison's disease is suspected (optional)

hypothyroidism, Addison's disease and diabetes mellitus. The prevalence of antibodies directed against the ovary has been the subject of significant research. Circulating anti-ovarian antibodies have been found in 10%–69% of women with POF but also in a significant number of controls. Chromosome analysis is unlikely to reveal any abnormality since her children are normal. The diagnostic usefulness of ovarian biopsy outside the context of a research setting has yet to be proved.[3] No single test such as FSH, luteinizing hormone, oestradiol, inhibin B and anti-Mullerian hormone, total antral follicle count and ovarian volume are reliable in predicting ovarian reserve and fertility. A combination of markers ultimately may be more helpful. In the absence of risk factors for osteoporosis, bone mineral density is unlikely to be compromised since the patient is still menstruating and this measurement can be deferred.

What are the long-term health implications?

Women with untreated premature menopause are at increased risk of developing osteoporosis and cardiovascular disease but at lower risk of breast malignancy.[4–7] Mean life expectancy in women with menopause before the age of 40 years is 2.0 years shorter than that in women with menopause after the age of 55 years. Premature menopause can lead to reduced peak bone mass (if the woman is younger than 25 years) or early bone loss thereafter. The increased risk of coronary heart disease has been noted especially in smokers.

What treatment should you recommend?

Patients must be provided with adequate information. She may find it a difficult diagnosis to accept, especially if she wishes to have further children.[8] National self-support groups for POF exist and these provide helpful psychological support for many women.

Oestrogen replacement therapy is the mainstay of treatment for women with POF and is recommended until the average age of natural menopause. This view is endorsed by national and international regulatory bodies. There is no evidence that oestrogen replacement increases the risk of breast cancer to a level greater than that found in normally menstruating women, and women with POF do not need to start mammographic screening early.[9] Hormone replacement therapy (HRT) or the combined oestrogen and progestogen contraceptive pill may be used. Women with POF who take HRT may need a higher dose of oestrogen to control vasomotor symptoms than women in their fifties.

However, this patient is using an intrauterine device for contraception. If she does not wish to have further children she may elect to change her device to the levonorgestrel-releasing intrauterine system (LNG-IUS) which would provide the progestogen component of her HRT. No clinical trial evidence attests the efficacy or safety of the use of non-oestrogen based treatments, such as bisphosphonates, strontium ranelate or raloxifene, in these women.

Some women complain of reduced libido or sexual function despite apparently adequate doses of oestrogen replacement. Testosterone should be considered and a testosterone patch for female use is now available.[10]

What are the fertility/contraception issues?

It is important to ascertain if the patient wishes to have further children or not. While women with premature menopause have traditionally been considered to be infertile, the lifetime chance of spontaneous conception in women with karyotypically normal POF has been estimated at 5%–15%. Donor oocyte *in vitro* fertilization would need to be discussed (see Case 19: Assisted Conception Methods). If she does not want to have further children she would need to consider continuing an effective form of contraception. The next decision will be how long she should continue with contraception. Traditionally, women have been advised that contraception can be stopped if they have been amenorrhoeic for two years before the age of 50 years and one year above that. However, her menstrual pattern will be difficult to establish if she is using HRT and she could be advised to continue with contraception until the age of 55 years.[11]

Recent Developments

As well as increasing the risk of cardiovascular disease and osteoporosis, early ovarian failure can have other health consequences. Oophorectomy performed before the onset of menopause for non-cancer indications increases the risk of cognitive impairment, dementia and parkinsonism.[12,13] While these findings need to be replicated in other studies this should be borne in mind when counselling women undergoing oophorectomy.

Conclusion

There has been some confusion about the management of premature ovarian failure among women and healthcare professionals since the publication of the Women's Health Initiative and the Million Women Study. Both studies were undertaken in women aged 50 and older and cannot be extrapolated to their younger counterparts. This is because younger women would normally be producing endogenous oestrogen because they have functioning ovaries. Oestrogen based replacement therapy is the mainstay of treatment for women with premature ovarian failure and is recommended at least until the average age of natural menopause (52 years in the UK). This view is endorsed by regulatory bodies such as the Committee on Safety of Medicines (now the Commission on Human Medicines) in the UK.

No evidence shows that oestrogen replacement increases the risk of breast cancer to a level greater than that found in normally menstruating women. Women with premature ovarian failure do not need to start mammographic screening early unless other risk factors are present, such as family history.

Further Reading

1 Pitkin J, Rees MCP, Gray S, Lumsden MA, Marsden J, Stevenson JC, Williamson J. British Menopause Society Council Consensus Statement. Management of premature menopause. *Menopause Int* 2007; **13**: 44–5.

2 Tucker D. Premature ovarian failure. In: Rees M, Hope S, Ravnikar V (eds). *The Abnormal Menstrual Cycle*. Abingdon: Taylor and Francis, 2005; 111–22.

3 Lutchman Singh K, Davies M, Chatterjee R. Fertility in female cancer survivors: pathophysiology, preservation and the role of ovarian reserve testing. *Hum Reprod Update* 2005; **11**: 69–89.

4 Rocca WA, Grossardt BR, de Andrade M, Malkasian GD, Melton LJ 3rd. Survival patterns after oophorectomy in premenopausal women: a population-based cohort study. *Lancet Oncol* 2006; **7**: 821–8.

5 Jacobsen BK, Knutsen SF, Fraser GE. Age at natural menopause and total mortality and mortality from ischemic heart disease: the Adventist Health Study. *J Clin Epidemiol* 1999; **52**: 303–7.

6 Ossewaarde ME, Bots ML, Verbeek AL, Peeters PH, van der Graaf Y, Grobbee DE, van der Schouw YT. Age at menopause, cause-specific mortality and total life expectancy. *Epidemiology* 2005; **16**: 556–62.

7 Titus-Ernstoff L, Longnecker MP, Newcomb PA, Dain B, Greenberg ER, Mittendorf R, Stampfer M, Willett W. Menstrual factors in relation to breast cancer risk. *Cancer Epidemiol Biomarkers Prev* 1998; **7**: 783–9.

8 Groff AA, Covington SN, Halverson LR, Fitzgerald OR, Vanderhoof V, Calis K, Nelson LM. Assessing the emotional needs of women with spontaneous premature ovarian failure. *Fertil Steril* 2005; **83**: 1734–41.

9 Ewertz M, Mellemkjaer L, Poulsen AH, Friis S, Sorensen HT, Pedersen L, McLaughlin JK, Olsen JH. Hormone use for menopausal symptoms and risk of breast cancer. A Danish cohort study. *Br J Cancer* 2005; **92**: 1293–7.

10 Shifren JL, Davis SR, Moreau M, Waldbaum A, Bouchard C, DeRogatis L, Derzko C, Bearnson P, Kakos N, O'Neill S, Levine S, Wekselman K, Buch A, Rodenberg C, Kroll R. Testosterone patch for the treatment of hypoactive sexual desire disorder in naturally menopausal women: results from the INTIMATE NM1 Study. *Menopause* 2006; **13**: 770–9.

11 Faculty of Family Planning and Reproductive Health Care. Clinical Effectiveness Unit. Contraception for women aged over 40 years. *J Fam Plann Reprod Health Care* 2005; **31**: 51–64.

12 Rocca WA, Bower JH, Maraganore DM, Ahlskog JE, Grossardt BR, de Andrade M, Melton LJ 3rd. Increased risk of cognitive impairment or dementia in women who underwent oophorectomy before menopause. *Neurology* 2007; **69**: 1074–83.

13 Rocca WA, Bower JH, Maraganore DM, Ahlskog JE, Grossardt BR, de Andrade M, Melton LJ 3rd. Increased risk of Parkinsonism in women who underwent oophorectomy before menopause. *Neurology* 2007; [Epub ahead of print].

13 Osteoporosis

Case History

A 56-year-old woman slipped on wet leaves whilst taking her chocolate Labrador for his walk, sustaining a Colles fracture. She had a premature menopause at the age of 38 years, but has only taken hormone replacement therapy (HRT) intermittently because of media scares about safety. She still has debilitating hot flushes. She has had a dual-energy X-ray absorptiometry (DEXA) scan and was found to be osteopenic with a T-score of –2.3 at the hip.

What hormonal treatment options would you advise?

What non-oestrogen based treatments are available?

How would you monitor treatment?

Background

Osteoporosis affects one in three women (see Case 44: Osteoporosis). Her major risk factor for osteoporosis is her premature menopause with intermittent use of hormone replacement therapy. A major concern is that having had one fracture she is likely to have another.[1] She also has vasomotor symptoms.

What hormonal treatment options would you advise?

Evidence from randomized controlled trials (including the Women's Health Initiative [WHI]) shows that HRT reduces the risk of spine and hip fractures, as well as other osteoporotic fractures.[2] While some studies show that a short duration of oestrogen use has long-term preventive effects on fracture, most epidemiological studies suggest that continuous and lifelong use is required for HRT to be an effective method of preventing fracture.[3] Regulatory authorities have advised that HRT should **not** be used as a first-line treatment for osteoporosis prevention, as the risks outweigh the benefits. This may be true for a population with no increased risk of osteoporosis (as in the WHI), but the risk–benefit ratio changes favourably when a population with increased risk of osteoporosis is targeted. Also HRT might be a first-line option for this patient since she also has hot flushes.[4] The 'standard' doses of oestrogen said to be bone-protective were oestradiol 1–2 mg, conjugated equine oestrogens 0.625 mg and transdermal 25–50 µg patch. However, lower doses may be protective. The relative risk of breast cancer on combined HRT is 2.17 after 5–9 years use, but women also need to realize that there is a similar doubling of risk with obesity (body mass index >30 kg/m^2) or drinking >3 units of alcohol per day.[5] Tibolone is classified as HRT in the United Kingdom British National Formulary. It conserves bone mass, and preliminary data have demonstrated a reduction in vertebral fractures. From the Million Women Study, the relative risk of breast cancer with tibolone is 1.45. Before prescribing HRT the woman must be aware of the full pros and cons of HRT and make her evidence-based patient choice, and her decision either way should be documented in the medical notes.

What non-oestrogen based treatments are available?

A variety of treatment options are available, but most have been studied in older women, few data exist about long-term efficacy in reducing fractures (i.e. ten years or more of treatment) and none will improve this woman's hot flushes. All interventions except for parathyroid hormone and strontium ranelate act mainly by inhibiting bone resorption (Table 13.1). In all studies the 'placebo' group received calcium and vitamin D supplements, and all 'active' groups received calcium and vitamin D augmentation if they were deficient, so co-prescribing with calcium and vitamin D must not be forgotten if it is likely that she is deficient.

Bisphosphonates

Alendronate, risedronate, etidronate and ibandronate are used in the prevention and treatment of osteoporosis. Bisphosphonates can be classified into two groups:

- non-nitrogen-containing bisphosphonates, such as etidronate

- nitrogen-containing bisphosphonates, such as alendronate, risedronate and ibandronate.

Table 13.1 Non-oestrogen based treatments for the prevention and treatment of osteoporosis

	Spine	Hip
Bisphosphonates		
Etidronate	A	B
Alendronate	A	A
Risedronate	A	A
Ibandronate	A	ND
Calcitriol	A	ND
Calcitonin	A	B
Selective oestrogen receptor modulators (SERMs)	A	ND
Strontium ranelate	A	A
Teriparatide / Preotact (1–84)(parathyroid hormone)	A	ND

ND = not demonstrated

The levels of evidence for the various agents detailed are:

A = meta-analysis of randomized controlled trials (RCTs) or from at least one RCT or from at least one well-designed controlled study without randomization

B = from at least one other type of well-designed quasi-experimental study or from well-designed non-experimental descriptive studies (e.g. comparative studies, correlation studies and case–control studies)

Alendronate and risedronate reduce the risk of vertebral and non-vertebral fractures, including hip fractures, and are considered first-line options for preventing post-menopausal osteoporosis.[4,6] All bisphosphonates are absorbed poorly from the gastro-intestinal tract and must be given on an empty stomach. Food or calcium-containing drinks (except water) inhibit the absorption, which at best is only 5%–10% of the admin-istered dose. The principal side effect of all bisphosphonates is irritation of the upper gastrointestinal tract. Symptoms resolve quickly after drug withdrawal and these adverse effects are much reduced by using weekly or monthly rather than daily regimens, but about 30% of patients give up bisphosphonates due to gastrointestinal side effects.

An intravenous formulation of ibandronate is approved for post-menopausal osteo-porosis. It is given as an injection over 15–30 seconds every three months. Antifracture efficacy has not been directly shown for this formulation or for the oral 150 mg once-monthly regimen, but it is assumed from a bridging study based on changes in bone min-eral density (BMD).

The question of how long to prescribe a bisphosphonate has not yet been fully clarified because of concerns about 'frozen bone', with complete turning-off of bone remodelling with long-term use and also development of osteonecrosis in the jaw, especially using intravenous preparations with people undergoing chemotherapy. However osteonecro-sis of the jaw is rarely associated with oral bisphosphonates used to treat osteoporosis.[6,7] Comparisons have been made between alendronate and risedronate, and between alen-dronate and raloxifene, but so far they have been mainly limited to their effects on BMD rather than the risk of fracture.[8] Randomized trials are required.

It is possible that the maximal benefit is derived from alendronate in five years of treat-ment, and then stopping, but it is not certain how to monitor these women until serum measurements of bone markers are more widespread and reliable.

Selective oestrogen receptor modulators

Compounds that possess oestrogenic actions in certain tissues and anti-oestrogenic actions in others are described as Selective oEstrogen Receptor Modulators, or SERMs. Raloxifene is licensed for the prevention of osteoporosis-related vertebral fracture. It does not help menopausal symptoms but gives the woman hot flushes, and although it reduces vertebral fractures (by about 30%) it does not prevent hip fractures. It does, however, reduce the breast cancer risk by a third in osteoporotic women. New SERMS that are undergoing phase III trials are awaited.

Parathyroid hormone peptides

Although hyperparathyroidism is associated with bone loss, the interaction between the peptide parathyroid hormone (PTH), which contains 84 amino acids, and the skeleton is more complex than was initially thought. Although continuous or tonic production of PTH promotes osteoclastic bone resorption, pulsed or clonic release of hormone seems to have precisely the opposite effect. There are two preparations. Recombinant 1-34 parathyroid hormone is given as a subcutaneous daily injection of 20 μg. The full 1-84 parathyroid hormone peptide is given in the same way in a daily dose of 100 μg. They reduce vertebral but not hip fractures in post-menopausal women with osteoporosis, but not hip fractures. Because they cost more than other options, they are reserved for patients with severe osteoporosis who are unable to tolerate or seem to be unresponsive to other treatments.

Strontium ranelate

Randomized controlled trials have shown a decreased risk of vertebral and hip fractures with strontium ranelate treatment. There are good data for the elderly (age >80 years) showing a reduction in hip and vertebral fractures within a year.[9] A 2 g sachet is administered daily, with the sachet's contents dissolved in water; it should be taken at least two hours after food. The most common side effects are mild and transient nausea and diarrhoea but are rare in absolute terms, and strontium is well tolerated. There is a slight, unexplained increased risk of venous thromboembolism, so it should be used with caution in women with a proven venous thromboembolism.

Calcitriol and calcitonin

Calcitriol is the active metabolite of vitamin D and facilitates the intestinal absorption of calcium. The potential dangers of hypercalcaemia and hypercalciuria mean that levels of calcium in serum and urine should be monitored closely, so use of calcitriol is limited.[10]

Calcitonin can be given by subcutaneous or intramuscular injection or by nasal spray. Parenteral calcitonin is expensive, produces side effects such as nausea, diarrhoea and flushing and results in the production of neutralizing antibodies in some patients. Nasal calcitonin has also been shown to reduce new vertebral fractures in women with established osteoporosis. An oral preparation is being developed.

How would you monitor treatment?

Whether treatment response should be monitored and, if so, whether bone density measurements or biochemical markers should be used, is unclear.[11] There is some variation among the guidelines with regard to the frequency of repeat measurements. In the United States, most private healthcare plans provide coverage for BMD testing to monitor the therapeutic response to therapy, but they generally will not reimburse testing for this indication more often than every two years.[11] It should be noted that, because of its higher atomic weight, strontium attenuates X-rays more strongly than calcium, leading to overestimated X-ray absorptiometry measurements of BMD.[12] While corrections have been calculated, they need further assessment. Biochemical markers of bone turnover are particularly attractive as a means of monitoring therapeutic efficacy because significant suppression of bone turnover occurs far more rapidly than detectable changes in BMD. They reach a nadir within three to six months of initiation of therapy in clinical trials. However, the imprecision of measuring bone turnover using markers is far greater than that of measuring BMD using DEXA, and cut-off values for the use of markers of bone turnover are uncertain.

Recent Developments

1   New treatments are being explored to expand the armamentarium for osteoporosis. Yearly intravenous bisphosphonates are being studied. A randomized placebo-controlled trial of yearly zoledronic acid first administered within 90 days after surgical repair of a hip fracture found that the rates of any new clinical fracture were 8.6% in the zoledronic acid group and 13.9% in the

placebo group. No cases of osteonecrosis of the jaw were reported, and no adverse effects on the healing of fractures were noted.[13]

2   The discovery of receptor activator of nuclear factor-kappaB ligand (RANKL) as a pivotal regulator of osteoclast activity provides a new therapeutic target. Early studies have demonstrated that denosumab, an investigational, highly specific anti-RANKL antibody, rapidly and substantially reduces bone resorption. Pharmacokinetics of the antibody allow dosing by subcutaneous injection at an interval of 6 months. Inhibiting RANKL appears to be a promising new treatment for osteoporosis and related disorders. More information about the effectiveness of denosumab in reducing fracture risk, its tolerability and safety, and the response to discontinuing therapy will be provided by ongoing clinical studies.[14]

3   Maintaining a healthy lifestyle through diet and exercise are also important. Tai Chi has been evaluated in a systematic review as an intervention to reduce rate of bone loss in post-menopausal women. Six controlled studies were identified. There were two RCTs, two non-randomized prospective parallel cohort studies, and two cross-sectional studies. The two RCTs and one of the prospective cohort studies suggested that Tai Chi-naive women who participated in Tai Chi training exhibited reduced rates of post-menopausal decline in BMD. Cross-sectional studies suggested that long-term Tai Chi practitioners had higher BMD than age-matched sedentary controls, and had slower rates of post-menopausal BMD decline. No adverse effects related to Tai Chi were reported in any trial. The authors concluded that this limited evidence suggests Tai Chi may be an effective, safe, and practical intervention for maintaining BMD in post-menopausal women.[15]

Conclusion

Osteoporosis is common. If she is symptomatic she would do well taking systemic HRT. Non-oestrogen based treatments will reduce fracture risk but not deal with menopausal symptoms.

Further Reading

1   Center JR, Bliuc D, Nguyen TV, Eisman JA. Risk of subsequent fracture after low-trauma fracture in men and women. *JAMA* 2007; **297**: 387–94.

2   Cauley JA, Robbins J, Chen Z, Cummings SR, Jackson RD, LaCroix AZ, LeBoff M, Lewis CE, McGowan J, Neuner J, Pettinger M, Stefanick ML, Wactawski-Wende J, Watts NB; Women's Health Initiative Investigators. Effects of estrogen plus progestin on risk of fracture and bone mineral density: the Women's Health Initiative randomized trial. *JAMA* 2003; **290**: 1729–38.

3   Bagger YZ, Tanko LB, Alexandersen P, Hansen HB, Mollgaard A, Ravn P, Qvist P, Kanis JA, Christiansen C. Two to three years of hormone replacement treatment in healthy women have long-term preventive effects on bone mass and osteoporotic fractures: the PERF study. *Bone* 2004; **34**: 728–35.

4 Poole KE, Compston JE. Osteoporosis and its management. *BMJ* 2006; **333**: 1251–6.

5 Beral V; Million Women Study Collaborators. Breast cancer and hormone-replacement therapy in the Million Women Study. *Lancet* 2003; **362**: 419–27.

6 Silverman SL, Maricic M. Recent developments in bisphosphonate therapy. *Semin Arthritis Rheum* 2007; **37**: 1–12.

7 Basu N, Reid DM. Bisphosphonates and osteonecrosis of the jaw. *Menopause Int* 2007; **13**: 56–9.

8 Silverman SL, Watts NB, Delmas PD, Lange JL, Lindsay R. Effectiveness of bisphosphonates on nonvertebral and hip fractures in the first year of therapy: the risedronate and alendronate (REAL) cohort study. *Osteoporos Int* 2007; **18**: 25–34.

9 Reginster JY, Malaise O, Neuprez A, Bruyere O. Strontium ranelate in the prevention of osteoporotic fractures. *Int J Clin Pract* 2007; **61**: 324–8.

10 Rees M, Purdie DW (eds). *Management of the Menopause: The Handbook*, 4th edn. London: Royal Society of Medicine Press, 2006.

11 Bonnick SL, Shulman L. Monitoring osteoporosis therapy: bone mineral density, bone turnover markers, or both? *Am J Med* 2006; **119** (4 Suppl 1): S25–31.

12 Blake GM, Fogelman I. Effect of bone strontium on BMD measurements. *J Clin Densitom* 2007; **10**: 34–8.

13 Lyles KW, Colon-Emeric CS, Magaziner JS, Adachi JD, Pieper CF, Mautalen C, Hyldstrup L, Recknor C, Nordsletten L, Moore KA, Lavecchia C, Zhang J, Mesenbrink P, Hodgson PK, Abrams K, Orloff JJ, Horowitz Z, Eriksen EF, Boonen S; the HORIZON Recurrent Fracture Trial. Zoledronic Acid and Clinical Fractures and Mortality after Hip Fracture. *N Engl J Med* 2007; [Epub ahead of print].

14 McClung M. Role of RANKL inhibition in osteoporosis. *Arthritis Res Ther* 2007; **9** (Suppl 1): S3.

15 Wayne PM, Kiel DP, Krebs DE, Davis RB, Savetsky-German J, Connelly M, Buring JE. The effects of Tai Chi on bone mineral density in postmenopausal women: a systematic review. *Arch Phys Med Rehabil* 2007; **88**: 673–80.

14 Post-menopausal Bleeding

Case History

A 54-year-old patient complains of post-menopausal bleeding (PMB) for a 'few months'. She is not on hormone replacement therapy (HRT) and her last menstrual period was over one year ago. Relevant features in her medical history are obesity and type 2 diabetes.

How do you clinically assess this patient?

Which is the most cost-effective triage for the evaluation of PMB?

Which endometrial thickness cut-off points are of significance in PMB?

When do you sample the endometrium in PMB?

How do you manage an initial negative investigation and persisting PMB?

Background

Post-menopausal bleeding (PMB) can be defined as (a) bleeding from the genital tract following at least six months of continuous amenorrhoea in menopausal women not on HRT or (b) breakthrough vaginal bleeding in post-menopausal women receiving HRT.

How do you clinically assess this patient?

The principal aim of investigation in PMB is to identify or exclude endometrial or cervical pathology, most notably endometrial cancer. The reported incidence of endometrial cancer in patients with PMB ranges from 9% to 12%. The probability of cancer as the underlying cause of PMB is age-dependent and increases from 9% for patients in their 50s to 60% for those in their 80s.[1] Although endometrial cancer and other cancers are significant conditions to exclude in PMB, the most common causes for PMB are non-malignant and include atrophic changes and HRT problems (Table 14.1).

If a woman presents with PMB it is important to take a history to establish (a) if there are any risk factors associated with endometrial cancer (e.g. obesity, diabetes) and (b) if the reason for the bleeding in a woman taking HRT might be caused by poor compliance, poor gastrointestinal absorption (e.g. gastroenteritis) or drug interactions. An abdominal and pelvic examination is mandatory in all women complaining of PMB, as vulvar or vaginal lesions, signs of trauma, and cervical polyps or other cervical abnormalities have to be excluded. This examination also gives the opportunity to take a routine cervical smear if this is appropriate.[2]

Table 14.1 Causes of post-menopausal bleeding	
Cause	Percentage
Atrophic endometritis	30%
Hormone replacement therapy	30%
Endometrial cancer	15%
Endometrial hyperplasia	10%
Endometrial or cervical polyps	10%
Other	5%
Source: Symonds 2001.[1]	

Which is the most cost-effective triage for the evaluation of PMB?

Transvaginal ultrasound scanning (TVS) has become the gold standard for the initial non-invasive assessment of PMB (Figure 14.1). It measures endometrial thickness and will also give information on other pelvic pathology such as fibroids and ovarian cysts. TVS-initiated triage has substantial cost savings versus biopsy-based algorithms in evaluating typical populations of post-menopausal women with abnormal vaginal bleeding.[3]

Which endometrial thickness cut-off points are of significance in PMB?

The interpretation of a TVS result in patients with PMB depends on the probability of the patient having cancer. The probability depends on her history of HRT, her age and other risk factors such as tamoxifen use or having a family history of endometrial cancer. Consequently, different endometrial thickness cut-off points have been applied to different groups of women with PMB: 3 mm, 4 mm and 5 mm.[4-7] An endometrial thickness of 3 mm or less gives a pre-test probability of cancer of 0.6% to 0.8% in (a) post-menopausal women who have never been on HRT, (b) post-menopausal women who have not been on any form of HRT for a year or more and (c) post-menopausal women on continuous combined HRT. In patients who present with unscheduled bleeding/PMB on sequential HRT, an endometrial thickness of 5 mm or less on TVS gives a probability of endometrial cancer of about 0.2%. Therefore in this subgroup of patients the 5 mm cut-off point provides reassurance that an endometrial cancer is unlikely to be present.

When do you sample the endometrium in PMB?

The finding of an endometrial thickness above the relevant cut-off point (3 mm or 5 mm) indicates that there is a risk of malignancy significant enough to warrant further investigation including an endometrial biopsy. There are two main techniques for endometrial biopsy: an aspiration curettage as an outpatient procedure and a dilatation and curettage (D&C) under anaesthetic. No existing method samples the entire uterine cavity. Therefore in most cases endometrial biopsy has to be complementary to other techniques, like a hysteroscopy, to increase sensitivity.

The advantage of aspiration curettage is that it avoids general anaesthetic and has fewer complications than D&C. However, entering the uterine cavity can be difficult and the degree of pain experienced may prevent obtaining a sample. Therefore aspiration

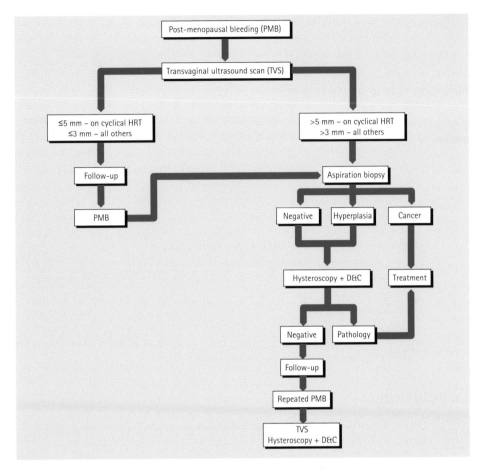

Figure 14.1 Algorithm for the management of post-menopausal bleeding.

curettage has a procedure failure rate as well as a tissue-yield failure rate, each of up to 10%. The two most commonly used devices are the Pipelle sampler and the Vabra curette. The Pipelle endometrial biopsy device was reported to have detection rates of 91% for endometrial carcinoma and atypical hyperplasia and to be superior to hysteroscopy and D&C.[8]

How do you manage an initial negative investigation and persisting PMB?

The classic method of obtaining endometrium is by D&C. However, as D&C is essentially a blind procedure it is estimated that in more than 50% of cases endometrial pathology is not uncovered.[9] Therefore, a D&C is commonly combined with a hysteroscopy, which allows direct visualization of the uterine cavity. There is general consensus that a hysteroscopy combined with a D&C is the current gold standard for endometrial sampling in PMB.[6] Consequently, a negative outpatient aspiration biopsy must be followed by a hysteroscopy and D&C. Similarly, a diagnosis of endometrial hyperplasia on aspiration biopsy does not obviate the need for further investigation, as hyperplasia may mask a carcinoma.

A dilemma exists if there is a negative initial endometrial sampling and PMB persists. Due to the high risk of a sampling error, which was reported to be up to 10%, a repeated TVS and biopsy is recommended in patients with persistent symptoms.[10]

Recent Developments

1 Patients' preferences for diagnostic management of PMB are also important.[11] This has been studied in a teaching hospital with office hysteroscopy facilities. The study found that most women wanted to be 100% certain that carcinoma could be ruled out. Only 5% of the women were willing to accept more than 5% risk of false reassurance. If the risk of recurrent bleeding due to benign disease exceeded 25%, the majority of women would prefer immediate diagnosis and treatment of benign lesions. This finding implies that the measurement of endometrial thickness with transvaginal ultrasound as a first-line test in the assessment of PMB should be reconsidered.

2 The offspring of women given diethylstilbestrol (DES) are now reaching the menopause. DES was given in an attempt to prevent multiple pregnancy-related problems such as miscarriage, premature birth, and abnormal bleeding. The recognition of the association of DES with an increased incidence of cervical and vaginal cancers in very young women led the Food and Drug Administration (FDA) to ban its use during pregnancy in 1971. It is not known how DES will affect the post-menopausal reproductive tract.[12]

Conclusion

Post-menopausal bleeding is a common reason for referral to a gynaecologist. Investigations should exclude malignancy and pre-malignancy, and diagnose the benign conditions that need treatment. This patient is at increased risk of endometrial cancer because of obesity and diabetes. Various countries have rapid access services for this problem.

Further Reading

1 Symonds I. Ultrasound, hysteroscopy and endometrial biopsy in the investigation of endometrial cancer. *Best Pract Res Clin Obstet Gynaecol* 2001; **15**: 381–91.

2 Oehler MK, MacKenzie I, Kehoe S, Rees MC. Assessment of abnormal bleeding in menopausal women: an update. *J Br Menopause Soc* 2003; **9**: 117–20.

3 Medverd JR, Dubinsky TJ. Cost analysis model: US versus endometrial biopsy in evaluation of peri- and postmenopausal abnormal vaginal bleeding. *Radiology* 2002; **222**: 619–27.

4 Gupta JK, Chien PF, Voit D, Clark TJ, Khan KS. Ultrasonographic endometrial thickness for diagnosing endometrial pathology in women with postmenopausal bleeding: a meta-analysis. *Acta Obstet Gynecol Scand* 2002; **81**: 799–816.

5 Weber AM, Belinson JL, Bradley LD, Piedmonte MR. Vaginal ultrasonography versus endometrial biopsy in women with postmenopausal bleeding. *Am J Obstet Gynecol* 1997; **177**: 924–9.

6 Scottish Intercollegiate Guidelines Network. Investigation of post-menopausal bleeding. Guideline No. 61. www.sign.ac.uk (accessed 20 09 07)

7 Granberg S, Ylostalo P, Wikland M, Karlsson B. Endometrial sonographic and histologic findings in women with and without hormonal replacement therapy suffering from postmenopausal bleeding. *Maturitas* 1997; **27**: 35–40.

8 Dijkhuizen FP, Mol BW, Brolmann HA, Heintz AP. The accuracy of endometrial sampling in the diagnosis of patients with endometrial carcinoma and hyperplasia: a meta-analysis. *Cancer* 2000; **89**: 1765–72.

9 Bettocchi S, Ceci O, Vicino M, Marello F, Impedovo L, Selvaggi L. Diagnostic inadequacy of dilatation and curettage. *Fertil Steril* 2001; **75**: 803–5.

10 Feldman S, Shapter A, Welch WR, Berkowitz RS. Two-year follow-up of 263 patients with post/perimenopausal vaginal bleeding and negative initial biopsy. *Gynecol Oncol* 1994; **55**: 56–9.

11 Timmermans A, Opmeer BC, Veersema S, Mol BW. Patients' preferences in the evaluation of postmenopausal bleeding. *BJOG* 2007; **114**: 1146–9.

12 Troisi R, Hatch EE, Titus-Ernstoff L, Hyer M, Palmer JR, Robboy SJ, Strohsnitter WC, Kaufman R, Herbst AL, Hoover RN. Cancer risk in women prenatally exposed to diethylstilbestrol. *Int J Cancer* 2007; **121**: 356–60.

PROBLEM

15 Menopausal Symptoms in Women with Breast Cancer

Case History

A 56-year-old woman comes complaining of hot flushes and vaginal dryness. She had a lumpectomy, radiotherapy and tamoxifen for an oestrogen receptor–positive invasive breast tumour six years ago and has not had a period for five years.

What are the issues?

What non-oestrogen based therapies can she use to control her flushes?

What can she use for vaginal dryness?

Background

What are the issues?

Breast cancer is a common condition and 212 920 women were expected to develop the disease in the United States in 2006.[1] Standard advice is to avoid systemic oestrogen (hormone replacement therapy [HRT]), especially in women with oestrogen receptor–positive tumours. Most clinical studies of patients with breast cancer who have been prescribed systemic oestrogens have not shown an adverse effect on survival; however, these studies involved small numbers of patients with short-term follow-up. The situation has become confused with the contradictory results of two randomized trials in Scandinavia (HABITS and Stockholm studies).[2,3] The HABITS study found an increased risk for women exposed to HRT but the Stockholm study did not. The increased risk of recurrence of breast cancer reported in HABITS has been suggested to be explained by the fact that most women randomized to HRT did not use concurrent tamoxifen and most used continuous combined HRT, whereas in the Stockholm study most women took tamoxifen and had long-cycle combined HRT. Thus, currently, the effect of HRT in women with breast cancer is uncertain.

What non-oestrogen based therapies can she use to control her flushes?

Pharmacological alternatives for hot flushes

Clonidine

Clonidine is a centrally acting α-adrenoceptor agonist that was developed originally for the treatment of hypertension. An oral dose of 50–75 µg twice daily has been used to treat vasomotor symptoms (Table 15.1). However, despite its popularity, evidence of efficacy in randomized controlled trials is poor.[4]

β-blockers

β-blockers have been postulated as a possible option for treating vasomotor symptoms, but results from the small trials which have been conducted have been disappointing.

Selective serotonin reuptake inhibitors (SSRIs) and serotonin and noradrenaline reuptake inhibitors (SNRIs)

Fluoxetine, paroxetine, citalopram and venlafaxine have been found to be effective in several studies. However most are short-lasting and effective only for a few weeks.[4] A nine-month placebo-controlled study of citalopram and fluoxetine showed no benefit for hot flushes.[5] The main drawback with these preparations is the high incidence of nausea, which often leads to withdrawal from therapy before maximum symptom-relief efficacy has been achieved. No studies evaluating the effect of SSRIs on sexuality in women with a history of breast cancer have been done either, although one of the side effects of these drugs is sexual dysfunction. Because hot flushes appear to have a negative effect on sexuality as well, problems in sexual functioning may well be aggravated with the use of SSRIs.

Gabapentin

Gabapentin is a gamma-aminobutyric acid analogue used to treat epilepsy, neurogenic pain and migraine. Again, evidence of efficacy for menopausal symptoms is poor and limited to short-term studies. The side effects most frequently seen in studies using gabapentin for the treatment of seizures include somnolence, dizziness, ataxia and fatigue.

Progestogens

Progestogens, such as 40 mg/day megestrol acetate or 5 mg/day norethisterone, can be effective in controlling hot flushes and night sweats.[6] However, at doses that achieve control of vasomotor symptoms, the risk of venous thromboembolism is increased.[7] Despite the effectiveness of progestogens for the treatment of hot flushes, there is a hesitation to use a hormonal agent in breast cancer patients, even though megestrol acetate has been used as a palliative agent for the disease. Irrefutable data that progestogens enhance the risk of breast cancer recurrence are lacking.

Tibolone

Tibolone is a synthetic steroid which is itself inert but after absorption is converted to metabolites with oestrogenic, progestogenic and androgenic actions. It is a 'no bleed' HRT and would be potentially suitable for this patient since she is post-menopausal. The daily dose is 2.5 mg. Preliminary analysis of the randomized LIBERATE trial of tibolone in breast cancer survivors has shown no adverse effects.[8] However, further data on breast cancer recurrence are required before recommending tibolone for this patient.

Table 15.1	Pharmacological and non-pharmacological options for treating menopausal symptoms in women with breast cancer	
Pharmacological	**Non-pharmacological**
SSRIs and SNRIs: fluoxetine, paroxetine, citalopram and venlafaxine	Diet and lifestyle
Gabapentin	Vaginal bioadhesive moisturizers
Clonidine	Vaginal lubricants
Progestogens	
Tibolone	
Vaginal oestradiol/oestriol	

Non-pharmacological

There is some evidence that more physically active women tend to suffer less from the symptoms of the menopause. Not all types of activity lead to an improvement in symptoms.[9] High-impact infrequent exercise may make symptoms worse; the best activity is aerobic, sustained regular exercise (e.g. swimming or running). Avoidance or reduction of intake of alcohol and caffeine can reduce the severity and frequency of vasomotor symptoms. Herbal products are best avoided because of potential oestrogenic actions (see Case 17: Alternative and Complementary Therapies for the Menopause).

What can she use for vaginal dryness?

Lubricants and vaginal moisturizers may help, but published data from scientific trials are limited.[10]

Lubricants are used mainly during intercourse and only have a temporary effect. Most are a combination of protectants and thickening agents in a water-soluble base. Lubricants must be applied frequently for more continuous relief and require reapplication before sexual activity. The integrity and efficacy of condoms may be compromised by lubricants such as petroleum-based products and baby oil. This is important when condoms are used to prevent sexually transmitted infections.

Moisturizers claim to provide a more long-lasting effect. They may contain a bioadhesive polycarbophil-based polymer, which attaches to mucin and epithelial cells on the vaginal wall and retains water. Moisturizers are promoted as providing long-term relief of vaginal dryness and need to be applied less frequently than lubricants.

Low-dose vaginal oestradiol and oestriol using the recommended doses are not contraindicated since systemic absorption is extremely low. They have the advantage of providing long-term relief and do not require application before sexual activity.

Recent Developments

1   Desvenlafaxine succinate (DVS) is a novel SNRI in clinical development for the treatment of menopausal hot flushes and, separately, for the treatment of major depressive disorder. Studies in animal models and in humans suggest that this may be a new therapeutic tool.[11]
2   Levetiracetam is an anti-epileptic agent that enhances GABAergic neurotransmission. A four-week pilot trial suggests that levetiracetam might be an effective therapy for the treatment of hot flushes.[12]

Conclusion

As survival from breast cancer is improving, maintaining quality of life is becoming an increasingly important issue. This patient elects for a trial of venlafaxine and low-dose vaginal oestrogens.

Further Reading

1   American Cancer Society. Cancer Facts & Figures 2006. www.cancer.org
2   Holmberg L, Anderson H. HABITS (hormonal replacement therapy after breast cancer—is it safe?), a randomised comparison: trial stopped. *Lancet* 2004; **363**: 453–5.
3   von Schoultz E, Rutqvist LE. Menopausal hormone therapy after breast cancer: the Stockholm randomized trial. *J Natl Cancer Inst* 2005; **97**: 533–5.
4   Albertazzi P. Noradrenergic and serotonergic modulation to treat vasomotor symptoms. *J Br Menopause Soc* 2006; **12**: 7–11.
5   Carpenter JS, Storniolo AM, Johns S, Monahan PO, Azzouz F, Elam JL, Johnson CS, Shelton RC. Randomized, double-blind, placebo-controlled crossover trials of venlafaxine for hot flashes after breast cancer. *Oncologist* 2007; **12**: 124–35.
6   Suvanto-Luukkonen E, Koivunen R, Sundström H, Bloigu R, Karjalainen E, Häivä-Mällinen L, Tapanainen JS. Citalopram and fluoxetine in the treatment of postmenopausal symptoms: a prospective, randomized, 9-month, placebo-controlled, double-blind study. *Menopause* 2005; **12**: 18–26.

7 Loprinzi CL, Michalak JC, Quella SK, O'Fallon JR, Hatfield AK, Nelimark RA, Dose AM, Fischer T, Johnson C, Klatt NE, *et al.* Megestrol acetate for the prevention of hot flashes. *N Engl J Med* 1994; **331**: 347–52.

8 Kroiss R, Fentiman IS, Helmond FA, Rymer J, Foidart JM, Bundred N, Mol-Arts M, Kubista E. The effect of tibolone in postmenopausal women receiving tamoxifen after surgery for breast cancer: a randomised, double-blind, placebo-controlled trial. *BJOG* 2005; **112**: 228–33.

9 Lindh-Astrand L, Nedstrand E, Wyon Y, Hammar M. Vasomotor symptoms and quality of life in previously sedentary postmenopausal women randomised to physical activity or estrogen therapy. *Maturitas* 2004; **48**: 97–105.

10 Bygdeman M, Swahn ML. Replens versus dienoestrol cream in the symptomatic treatment of vaginal atrophy in postmenopausal women. *Maturitas* 1996; **23**: 259–63.

11 Deecher DC, Alfinito PD, Leventhal L, Cosmi S, Johnston GH, Merchenthaler I, Winneker R. Alleviation of thermoregulatory dysfunction with the new serotonin and norepinephrine reuptake inhibitor desvenlafaxine succinate in ovariectomized rodent models. *Endocrinology* 2007; **148**: 1376–83.

12 Thompson S, Bardia A, Tan A, Barton DL, Kottschade L, Sloan JA, Christensen B, Smith D, Loprinzi CL. Levetiracetam for the treatment of hot flashes: a phase II study. *Support Care Cancer* 2007; [Epub ahead of print].

PROBLEM

16 Venous Thromboembolism

Case History

A 55-year-old woman comes complaining of severe hot flushes keeping her awake day and night. She is concerned in that she was told that she could not take hormone replacement therapy (HRT) because she was said to have suffered a deep vein thrombosis when taking the combined oral contraceptive (COC) pill when she was 25 years old. Her doctor told her to stop the pill and to rest. She subsequently had two uneventful pregnancies and was not anticoagulated.

What are the issues?

How do you assess the patient?

What are the management strategies?

Background

What are the issues?

Until 1996, when observational studies were published, HRT, unlike the combined oral contraceptive pill, was not suspected to increase the risk of venous thromboembolism (VTE).[1] Although HRT reduces fibrinogen and increases the natural anticoagulant protein C, it also decreases the natural anticoagulants antithrombin and protein S and increases factors VII and VIII and von Willebrand factor. Thus, the overall effect is to increase the tendency to VTE.[2,3] The best evidence comes from the randomized Heart and Estrogen/progestin Replacement Study (HERS) and Women's Health Initiative (WHI) studies.[4,5] For combined therapy, the odds ratio (OR) was 2.7 (95% confidence interval [CI] 1.4–5.0) in HERS and 2.1 (1.6–2.7) in WHI. These ORs are slightly lower than those for the second-generation COCs. The highest risk occurs in the first year of use. The absolute risk is small, however, as VTE occurs in 1.7 per 1000 in women older than 50 years who are not taking HRT and mortality is low (1%–2%). Advancing age, obesity and an underlying thrombophilia, such as Factor V Leiden, significantly increase risk. For example, in the placebo arm of the WHI study, the number of cases of VTE per 1000 women per year was 0.8 at age 50–59 years, 1.9 at 60–69 years and 2.7 at 70–79 years.

A proven history of VTE is the biggest risk factor for future events and is a relative contraindication to oestrogen-based HRT. After a single episode of VTE there is a constant risk of recurrence of 5% per year after anticoagulation is stopped. Most episodes of recurrence occur within the first year.

In women who have taken HRT after VTE, data from randomized trials show an increased risk of recurrence in the first year that the hormone is used.[6] Limited data suggest that transdermal HRT seems to be associated with a lower risk than oral therapy.[7,8]

How do you assess the patient?

It is essential to assess whether the deep vein thrombosis was confirmed objectively or not. From this history given by the patient it appears that she has been erroneously given the label of having had a VTE since she does not appear to have had any objective tests or treatment. It is reassuring that she had uncomplicated pregnancies. It is necessary to check the original medical notes to confirm the patient's recall of events, though this may be difficult after 30 years. If she was anticoagulated for several weeks, it would be prudent to consider the event confirmed. It would also be helpful to obtain a family history of episodes of VTE. A thrombophilia screen may then be undertaken, especially as there is some doubt about the diagnosis, as the finding of a severe defect or a combination of defects might alter the perceived risk–benefit assessment of giving HRT. However, a negative thrombophilia screen must not be used to give false reassurance in the presence of a family history of VTE, especially if unprovoked.

1 Take and check the personal history

2 Take a family history

3 Thrombophilia screen including genetic testing for Factor V Leiden and prothrombin mutation

What are the management strategies?

If a decision to use HRT is made, limited evidence suggests that the transdermal route might be safer than oral therapy. Occasionally, it is suggested that a women is anticoagulated to allow HRT to be given. It has to be appreciated that about 1 in 400 patients on warfarin bleed to death each year, so this is rarely the best option. As raloxifene and progestogens at doses higher than those used for contraceptive purposes increase the risk of VTE, these are probably best avoided.[9] The data for tibolone are uncertain. The effects of herbal therapies on coagulation are unknown. If she wishes to avoid hormonal therapies she could try a selective serotonin reuptake inhibitor (see Case 15: Menopausal Symptoms in Women with Breast Cancer).

Recent Developments

The effects of tibolone on VTE are uncertain since there are no large clinical trials as yet. Some experimental data suggest that tibolone may not have the same prothrombotic effects as oestrogen-based HRT.[10] Further research is required, however, before definite conclusions can be reached about the risk of VTE with tibolone.

It is now becoming apparent that different progestogens have varying effects on coagulation; norpregnane derivatives may be thrombogenic, whereas micronized progesterone and pregnane derivatives appear safe with respect to thrombotic risk.[11]

Conclusion

This case illustrates the dangers of giving labels to patients. It is most likely that she never had a deep vein thrombosis. If she elects to take HRT it is probably prudent to recommend transdermal oestrogen delivery.

Further Reading

1 Daly E, Vessey MP, Hawkins MM, Carson JL, Gough P, Marsh S. Risk of venous thromboembolism in users of hormone replacement therapy. *Lancet* 1996; **348**: 977–80.

2 Keeling DM. Hormone replacement therapy, thrombosis and thrombophilia. *J Br Menopause Soc* 2005; **11**: 74–5.

3 Royal College of Obstetricians and Gynaecologists (RCOG). *Hormone Replacement Therapy and Venous Thromboembolism*. Green-top Guideline No. 19. London: RCOG Press, 2004.

4 Grady D, Wenger NK, Herrington D, Khan S, Furberg C, Hunninghake D, Vittinghoff E, Hulley S. Postmenopausal hormone therapy increases risk for venous thromboembolic disease. The Heart and Estrogen/progestin Replacement Study. *Ann Intern Med* 2000; **132**: 689–96.

5 Cushman M, Kuller LH, Prentice R, Rodabough RJ, Psaty BM, Stafford RS, Sidney S, Rosendaal FR. Estrogen plus progestin and risk of venous thrombosis. *JAMA* 2004; **292**: 1573–80.

6 Høibraaten E, Qvigstad E, Arnesen H, Larsen S, Wickstrøm E, Sandset PM. Increased risk of recurrent venous thromboembolism during hormone replacement therapy – results of the randomized, double-blind, placebo-controlled estrogen in venous thromboembolism trial (EVTET). *Thromb Haemost* 2000; **84**: 961–7.

7 Scarabin PY, Oger E, Plu-Bureau G; EStrogen and THromboEmbolism Risk (ESTHER) Study Group. Differential association of oral and transdermal oestrogen-replacement therapy with venous thromboembolism risk. *Lancet* 2003; **362**: 428–32.

8 Canonico M, Oger E, Conard J, Meyer G, Levesque H, Trillot N, Barrellier MT, Wahl D, Emmerich J, Scarabin PY; EStrogen and THromboEmbolism Risk (ESTHER) Study Group. Obesity and risk of venous thromboembolism among postmenopausal women: differential impact of hormone therapy by route of estrogen administration. The ESTHER Study. *J Thromb Haemost* 2006; **4**: 1259–65.

9 Vasilakis C, Jick H, del Mar Melero-Montes M. Risk of idiopathic venous thromboembolism in users of progestagens alone. *Lancet* 1999; **354**: 1610–11.

10 Winkler UH, Altkemper R, Kwee B, Helmond FA, Coelingh Bennink HJ. Effects of tibolone and continuous combined hormone replacement therapy on parameters in the clotting cascade: a multicenter, double-blind, randomized study. *Fertil Steril* 2000; **74**: 10–19.

11 Canonico M, Oger E, Plu-Bureau G, Conard J, Meyer G, Levesque H, Trillot N, Barrellier MT, Wahl D, Emmerich J, Scarabin PY; Estrogen and Thromboembolism Risk (ESTHER) Study Group. Hormone therapy and venous thromboembolism among postmenopausal women: impact of the route of estrogen administration and progestogens: the ESTHER study. *Circulation* 2007; **115**: 840–5.

17 Alternative and Complementary Therapies for the Menopause

Case History

A 54-year-old woman comes complaining of hot flushes. She does not wish to take hormone replacement therapy (HRT) and wants to discuss alternative and complementary therapies.

What is available and what is the evidence of efficacy?

What are the safety issues?

Are there interactions with standard medication?

Background

Many women wish to use alternative and complementary therapies in the belief that they are safer and 'more natural' following media scares and uncertainties regarding oestrogen-based HRT.[1,2] Although individual trials suggest benefits from certain therapies (Table 17.1), data are insufficient to support the effectiveness of any complementary and alternative therapy for the management of menopausal symptoms.[3]

What is available and what is the evidence of efficacy?

Phyto-oestrogens

Phytoestrogens are plant substances that have effects similar to those of oestrogens. The role of phyto-oestrogens has stimulated considerable interest, as women from populations that consume a diet high in isoflavones, such as the Japanese, are reported to have

Table 17.1 Alternative and complementary therapies for the management of menopausal symptoms	
Type	Source/examples
Phyto-oestrogens	Soy, red clover
Herbal remedies	Black cohosh, oil of evening primrose, ginkgo biloba, wild yams
Hormonal	DHEA, progesterone transdermal creams
Mechanical	Acupuncture, reflexology
Other	Homeopathy

fewer hot flushes.[4,5] The most important groups are called isoflavones and lignans. The major isoflavones are genistein and daidzein. The major lignans are enterolactone and enterodiol. Isoflavones are found mainly in soybeans, chickpeas and red clover. Oilseeds such as flaxseed are rich in lignans, and lignans are also found in cereal bran, whole cereals, vegetables, legumes and fruit. The evidence from randomized placebo-controlled trials for soy and derivatives of red clover is conflicting.[6]

Herbal remedies

A wide variety of herbal remedies exist but little is known about efficacy, safety and toxicity.

Black cohosh is used widely to alleviate menopausal symptoms. Results from placebo-controlled trials or comparison with conjugated equine oestrogens are conflicting.[6]

Evening primrose oil is rich in gamma-linolenic acid. One small, placebo-controlled, randomized trial showed it to be ineffective for treating hot flushes.[1,2]

Dong quai is used commonly in traditional Chinese medicine. It was not found to be superior to placebo in a randomized trial.[1,2]

Ginkgo biloba is widely used, but little evidence shows that it improves menopausal symptoms.

Ginseng is used extensively in eastern Asia but randomized trial data do not show it to be superior to placebo.[1,2]

Other herbs. St John's wort, agnus castus, liquorice root, valerian root and wild yam cream are also popular, but again there is no good evidence for efficacy. Claims have been made that steroids (diosgenin) in wild yams can be converted in the body to progesterone, but this is biochemically impossible in humans.

Hormonal preparations

Dehydroepiandrosterone

Dehydroepiandrosterone (DHEA) is a steroid secreted by the adrenal cortex. Blood levels of DHEA fall with age in both sexes. In the United States it is classed as a food supplement. Currently no evidence shows that DHEA has any effect on hot flushes.

Progesterone transdermal creams

Progesterone gels and creams have been available for a number of years. There are two licensed gels: one for topical use on the breast and the other for vaginal use for endometrial protection. However these products are not available in all countries. Transdermal progesterone creams have been promoted for the treatment of menopausal symptoms but the data are poor.

'Mechanical'

The term 'mechanical' is used as these therapies do not involve ingestion or application of any agent. These therapies include acupuncture, reflexology, acupressure, Alexander technique, Ayurveda, osteopathy magnetism and Reiki. Little is known about their effect on menopausal symptoms and the limited data do not show an effect.

Homeopathy

Samuel Hahnemann (1755–1843), a German physician and scientist, was the first proponent of homeopathy. He postulated that the homoeopathic remedy acted through a vital force, stimulating a healing or self-regulating response. He then proposed the concept of minimum dose – the smallest amount of a substance that could be given to avoid side effects and yet would still bring about a healing response. Data from case histories, observational studies and a small number of randomized trials are encouraging, but more research is clearly needed.[1,2]

What are the safety issues?

There are concerns about hepatotoxicity as has been found with black cohosh and kava kava.[3] The latter has been suspended or withdrawn by some regulatory authorities. Nephrotoxicity has also been reported. Some preparations may contain oestrogenic compounds and this is of concern for women with hormone-dependent tumours. An increased number of breast cancer metastases has been found in mouse mammary tumour virus/Neu transgenic mice receiving black cohosh.[7] Furthermore, a five-year follow-up study of soy indicated that users were at a significantly increased risk for endometrial hyperplasia compared with placebo.[8] To avoid the side effects of progestogens, some women who take oestrogens use transdermal progesterone creams for endometrial protection. However, there is no good evidence that transdermal progesterone creams induce secretory changes or prevent mitotic activity in an oestrogen-primed endometrium.[2] Finally, there is little control over the quality of individual products and thus it is unusual to know what is actually present in an individual preparation or supplement. Moreover, some preparations may contain high levels of heavy metals such as arsenic, lead and mercury.[1]

Are there interactions with standard medication?

Patients are often unaware that herb–drug interactions can be potentially fatal and do not tell their physician that they are taking a herbal remedy.[9] Adverse events resulting from herb–drug interactions include bleeding when combined with warfarin or aspirin; hypertension, coma and mild serotonin syndrome when combined with selective serotonin reuptake inhibitors; and reduced efficacy of anti-epileptics. A survey of emergency department admissions showed that aspirin and warfarin were the most commonly involved drugs.[10] For example, ginkgo can cause bleeding when combined with warfarin or aspirin, high blood pressure when combined with a thiazide diuretic and even coma when combined with trazodone. Ginseng reduces the blood concentrations of alcohol and warfarin and can induce mania when used concomitantly with phenelzine. St John's wort reduces the blood concentrations of cyclosporin, midazolam, tacrolimus, amitriptyline, digoxin, warfarin and theophylline. Reduced concentrations of cyclosporin have led to organ rejection. It also causes serotonin syndrome when used in combination with selective serotonin reuptake inhibitors (for example, sertraline and paroxetine).

Recent Developments

Populations that consume a diet high in phytoestrogens are said to have lower rates of cardiovascular disease, osteoporosis, and breast, colon, endometrial, and ovarian cancers. PHYTOS, ISOHEART, and PHYTOPREVENT are EU studies examining the role of phyto-oestrogens in osteoporosis, heart disease, and cancer.[11-13] Further well-designed, randomized trials are needed to determine the role and safety of phyto-oestrogen supplements in menopausal women and people who have survived cancer.

Conclusion

The efficacy and safety of alternative and complementary therapies warrant further study in well-designed clinical trials. While there is a European Union Directive on traditional herbal medicinal products, this will not cover products bought by women elsewhere.

Further Reading

1 Rees M, Purdie DW (eds). *Management of the Menopause: The Handbook*, 4th edn. London: Royal Society of Medicine Press, 2006.

2 Rees M, Mander A (eds). *Managing the Menopause Without Oestrogen*. London: Royal Society of Medicine Press, 2004.

3 Nedrow A, Miller J, Walker M, Nygren P, Huffman LH, Nelson HD. Complementary and alternative therapies for the management of menopause-related symptoms: a systematic evidence review. *Arch Intern Med* 2006; **166**: 1453–65.

4 Balk E, Chung M, Chew P, Ip S, Raman G, Kupelnick B, Tatsioni A, Sun Y, Devine D, Lau J. Effects of soy on health outcomes. *Evid Rep Technol Assess (Summ)* 2005; **126**: 1–8.

5 Booth NL, Piersen CE, Banuvar S, Geller SE, Shulman LP, Farnsworth NR. Clinical studies of red clover (Trifolium pratense) dietary supplements in menopause: a literature review. *Menopause* 2006; **13**: 251–64.

6 Newton KM, Reed SD, LaCroix AZ, Grothaus LC, Ehrlich K, Guiltinan J. Treatment of vasomotor symptoms of menopause with black cohosh, multibotanicals, soy, hormone therapy, or placebo: a randomized trial. *Ann Intern Med* 2006; **145**: 869–79.

7 Workshop on the Safety of Black Cohosh in Clinical Studies. Bethesda, MD: National Center for Complementary and Alternative Medicine, National Institutes of Health Office of Dietary Supplements, 2004.

8 Unfer V, Casini ML, Costabile L, Mignosa M, Gerli S, Di Renzo GC. Endometrial effects of long-term treatment with phytoestrogens: a randomized, double-blind, placebo-controlled study. *Fertil Steril* 2004; **82**: 145–8.

9 Hu Z, Yang X, Ho PC, Chan SY, Heng PW, Chan E, Duan W, Koh HL, Zhou S. Herb–drug interactions: a literature review. *Drugs* 2005; **65**: 1239–82.

10 Taylor DM, Walsham N, Taylor SE, Wong L. Potential interactions between prescription drugs and complementary and alternative medicines among patients in the emergency department. *Pharmacotherapy* 2006; **26**: 634–40.

11 PHYTOS. www.ec.europa.eu/research/endocrine/pdf/qlk1-ct2000-00431-year1.pdf (accessed 20 09 07)

12 ISOHEART. www.isoheart.kvl.dk/ (accessed 20 09 07)

13 PHYTOPREVENT www.phytoprevent.org (accessed 20 09 07)

Fertility and Contraction

PROBLEM

18 Subfertility Investigations

Case History

A 32-year-old woman attends clinic along with her partner. She is worried that after twelve months of trying, she has not become pregnant. Her cycle is fairly regular (every 29–32 days). Her only significant medical history is an episode of pelvic inflammatory disease (PID) seven years ago. Her partner is aged 33 years and is fit and well.

What would you advise them about the timing of intercourse?

How would you counsel them about the likelihood of a spontaneous conception?

What factors in the history would prompt you to investigate early?

What are the appropriate and relevant investigations?

Background

Infertility may be defined as failure to conceive after two years despite frequent sexual intercourse. One in seven couples encounter problems with their fertility.[1]

What would you advise them about the timing of intercourse?

Questions as to the frequency of sexual intercourse should be asked. Intercourse every two or three days may improve the chance of spontaneous conception because sperm can survive for up to seven days in the female genital tract.[2] Regular intercourse rather than timed intercourse should be advised because timed intercourse has been found to be emotionally stressful for couples.

How would you counsel them about the likelihood of a spontaneous conception?

The couple should be informed that although 84% of people who are trying to conceive will do so in one year, the cumulative pregnancy rate after two years of trying is 92%.[3]

What factors in the history would prompt you to investigate early?

Current guidelines suggest that, for most couples, investigation into infertility should begin after two years.[1] There are, however, situations where early investigation is appropriate (Table 18.1).

Early investigation of tubal patency is appropriate in a woman with a history of pelvic inflammatory disease. It is also appropriate in women with specific risk factors for ovarian failure, such as previous chemotherapy during treatment for cancer. Other factors in the history that may prompt early investigation are a history of oligomenorrhoea, amenorrhoea or other clinical signs of polycystic ovary syndrome.

Female fertility is known to decline significantly with age, especially after 35 years of age. In addition, the success rates of assisted reproduction methods decline steadily with age.[4] Data have suggested that the average prevalence of infertility is 5.5% at ages 25–29 years, 9.4% at ages 30–34 and 19.7% at ages 35–39.[5] Thus, investigation after one year of infertility may be appropriate in women who are aged over 35 years.

Table 18.1 Reasons to prompt early referral for investigation into infertility

Maternal age >35 years
Previous pelvic inflammatory disease
Previous chemotherapy/radiotherapy
Oligomenorrhoea/amenorrhoea
Known polycystic ovary syndrome

What are the appropriate and relevant investigations?

Assessing semen quality

Semen analysis is an essential part of the initial investigations into subfertility in any couple. It is therefore useful to see both partners for consultation. Low sperm count can be identified as the only cause of infertility in about 20% of couples but it may be contributory in a further 25% of couples. Semen analysis should be referenced to World Health Organization (WHO) criteria (Table 18.2).[6] An abnormal result should be repeated as semen quality varies over time.

Table 18.2 WHO criteria for semen analysis[6]

Criteria	Parameters
Volume	2.0–5.0 ml
pH	7.2 to 7.8
Sperm concentration	20×10^6 per ml or more
Total sperm count	40×10^6 spermatozoa or more
Motility	50% or more with forward progression or 25% or more with rapid linear progression within 60 minutes after collection
Morphology	50% or more with normal morphology
Viability	75% or more live (i.e. excluding dye)
White blood cells	Fewer than 1×10^6 per ml
Zinc (total)	2.4 mol or more per ejaculate
Citric acid (total)	52 mol (10 mg) or more per ejaculate
Fructose (total)	13 mol or more per ejaculate

Source: World Health Organization, 1999.[6]

Assessing ovulation

Regular menstrual cycles usually indicate ovulation. Anovulation accounts for about 21% of female infertility.[7] Ovulation is best confirmed retrospectively by measuring serum progesterone in the mid-luteal phase.[8] This equates to day 21 of a 28-day cycle. Women with a prolonged cycle will need the test performed later in the cycle (e.g. day 30 of a 37-day cycle). Those with irregular menses need the test repeated twice-weekly from day 21 until the next menstrual period starts. A serum progesterone level of 30 nmol/l is suggestive of ovulation although laboratory values may vary. Ovulation occurs after luteinization of a mature follicle. Thus modern home urine tests which detect the luteinizing hormone (LH) surge can suggest when ovulation is about to occur.

Follicle-stimulating hormone (FSH) and LH levels should be assessed between day 2 and day 5 of a cycle. Low FSH and LH levels may be found in women who have anorexia nervosa, have lost significant weight or those who exercise excessively. Raised FSH is seen in premature ovarian failure. Again, laboratory reference ranges may vary but FSH greater than 10 IU/l is suggestive of decreased ovarian reserve and FSH greater than 25 IU/l is suggestive of premature ovarian failure. Raised LH is suggestive (but not diagnostic) of polycystic ovary syndrome. LH will also be raised in ovarian failure.

Assessing tubal patency

Tubal disease accounts for about 14% of female subfertility.[7] The standard methods for assessing tubal patency are the hysterosalpingogram (HSG) or laparoscopy and dye test. More recently, hysterosalpingography contrast sonography has been used.

HSG is a simple procedure with few complications; it is therefore the first-line investigation for most women in subfertility investigation. HSG cannot distinguish between tubal occlusion and tubal spasm and therefore is an unreliable indicator of tubal occlusion. It is,

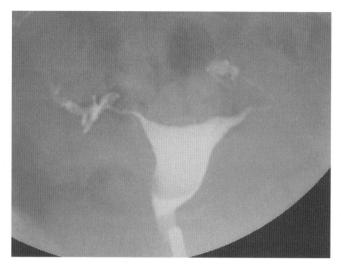

Figure 18.1 Hysterosalpingogram showing patent tubes.

however, a reliable indicator of tubal patency. When HSG suggests that the tubes are patent, this will be confirmed at laparoscopy in 94% of cases.[9] HSG should be performed in the first ten days of the cycle when there should be no risk of pregnancy (Figure 18.1).

Laparoscopy has the advantage of being able to assess the pelvis for other pathologies which may be associated with subfertility as well as assessing tubal patency. There is, however, significant morbidity associated with laparoscopy, such as the potential to damage the bladder or bowel.[10] Thus laparoscopy as a first-line investigation should be reserved for those women who are known or suspected to have other comorbidities such as endometriosis, previous ectopic pregnancy or PID.

Screening for infection

Chlamydia trachomatis is a common cause of PID which can lead to tubal factor infertility. Chlamydia infection is most common in the sexually active population under the age of 19 years. However the prevalence in subfertile women is only 1.9%.[11] Screening for chlamydia is still recommended because of the possibility of introduction or reactivation of infection at the time of uterine instrumentation at HSG or laparoscopy. Patients with a diagnosis of a sexually transmitted infection should be reviewed in a genitourinary medicine clinic so that full screening, treatment and contact tracing is assured.

Recent Developments

 The age-related decline of fertility is largely attributable to a progressive decline of ovarian responsiveness and oocyte quality and quantity. A number of so-called ovarian reserve tests (ORTs) have been designed to determine oocyte reserve and quality. These include early-follicular-phase blood values of FSH, oestradiol, inhibin B and anti-Müllerian hormone (AMH), the antral follicle count (AFC), the ovarian volume (OVVOL) and the ovarian blood flow, and furthermore the Clomiphene Citrate Challenge Test (CCCT), the exogenous FSH ORT (EFORT) and the gonadotrophin agonist stimulation test (GAST), all as measures to predict ovarian response and chance of pregnancy. In some centres many of these tests have become part of the routine diagnostic procedure for infertility patients who undergo assisted reproductive techniques. A systematic review of ORTs has shown that they have only modest-to-poor predictive properties.[12]

Conclusion

Infertility is a complicated, emotional and frustrating problem. Whilst adequate investigation should be offered, couples must be made aware that no cause may be found and assisted reproductive techniques may fail. Counselling therefore plays a key part in managing infertile couples.

Further Reading

1 National Institute for Health and Clinical Excellence. CG11 Fertility: Full guideline. February 2004. www.nice.org.uk/guidance/CG11/guidance/pdf/English (accessed 19 09 07)

2 Ferreira-Poblete A. The probability of conception on different days of the cycle with respect to ovulation: an overview. *Adv Contracep* 1997; **13**: 83–95.

3 van Noord-Zaadstra BM, Looman CWN, Alsbach H, Habbema JDF, te Velde ER, Karbaat J. Delaying childbearing: effect of age on fecundity and outcome of pregnancy. *BMJ* 1991; **302**: 1361–5.

4 The Human Fertility and Embryology Authority. www.hfea.gov.uk (accessed 19 09 07)

5 Bongaarts J. Infertility after age 30: a false alarm. *Fam Plann Perspect* 1982; **14**: 75–8.

6 World Health Organization. *WHO Laboratory Manual for the Examination of Human Semen and Sperm-cervical Mucus Interaction*, 4th edn. Cambridge: Cambridge University Press, 1999.

7 Hull MG, Glazener CM, Kelly NJ, Conway DI, Foster PA, Hinton RA, Coulson C, Lambert PA, Watt EM, Desai KM. Population study of causes, treatment, and outcome of infertility. *Br Med J (Clin Res Ed)* 1985; **291**: 1693–7.

8 Crosignani PG, Rubin BL. Optimal use of infertility diagnostic tests and treatments. The ESHRE Capri Workshop Group. *Hum Reprod* 2000; **15**: 723–32.

9 Swart P, Mol BW, van der Veen F, van Beurden M, Redekop WK, Bossuyt PM. The accuracy of hysterosalpingography in the diagnosis of tubal pathology: a meta-analysis. *Fertil Steril* 1995; **64**: 486–91.

10 Chapron C, Querleu D, Bruhat M, Madelenat P, Fernandez H, Pierre F, Dubuisson JB. Surgical complications of diagnostic and operative gynaecological laparoscopy: a series of 29,966 cases. *Hum Reprod* 1998; **13**: 867–72.

11 MacMillan S, Templeton A. Screening for *Chlamydia trachomatis* in subfertile women. *Hum Reprod* 1999; **14**: 3009–12.

12 Broekmans FJ, Kwee J, Hendriks DJ, Mol BW, Lambalk CB. A systematic review of tests predicting ovarian reserve and IVF outcome. *Hum Reprod Update* 2006; **12**: 685–718.

19 Assisted Conception Methods

Case History

A couple attend the fertility clinic. The female partner is 38 years old and has a regular 30-day cycle. Her luteal phase progesterone is suggestive of ovulation. Her partner has had a normal semen analysis. They have been trying to conceive for two years.

What methods of assisted conception are available?

Which surgical procedures might improve the chances of conception?

What irreversible factors would affect the outcome of assisted reproduction treatments?

Background

What methods of assisted conception are available?

Ovulation induction

Clomifene is an anti-oestrogen and is used to induce ovulation. It is associated with increased pregnancy rates per treatment cycle in patients with amenorrhoea and oligomenorrhoea.[1] It has also been shown to increase clinical pregnancy rates slightly in women with unexplained infertility.[2] The use of clomifene has about a 10% risk of multiple pregnancy; therefore ultrasound monitoring of the number of developing follicles must be offered, at least in the first cycle of treatment, to prevent the conception of high-order multiples. Gonadotrophins may also be used in clomifene-resistant women.

Intrauterine insemination (IUI)

Intrauterine insemination (Table 19.1) involves introducing prepared semen into the uterus. This can be done during the woman's own natural cycle, or as part of a stimulated cycle using clomifene or gonadotrophins. IUI has been shown to increase pregnancy rates in mild male factor infertility, unexplained subfertilty and subfertility related to minimal or mild endometriosis. Assuming that there are no complicating factors, such as a raised follicle-stimulating hormone (FSH), cumulative pregnancy rates may be as high as 35% after four cycles, particularly in male factor infertility.

Stimulated IUI carries with it a significant risk of multiple pregnancy and therefore unstimulated IUI is recommended.[3] Up to six cycles of IUI may be of benefit. However some patients, especially those who are older at initial presentation, will choose not to have IUI and to embark upon *in vitro* fertilization (IVF) instead, because of higher success rates per cycle.

Donor insemination

Donor insemination is a valuable method of assisted conception in cases of obstructive and non-obstructive azoospermia or very poor semen quality, where the couple do not wish to undergo IVF with intracytoplasmic sperm injection (ICSI). It can also be used to avoid transmission of inheritable diseases. Couples may choose to use donor insemination if attempts at ICSI have failed. Frozen semen which has been quarantined for six months is used rather than fresh semen to avoid transmission of diseases such as human immunodeficiency virus. Donors are tested for other sexually transmissible infections, as well as karyotyped for chromosomal abnormalities.

In vitro fertilization

Pregnancies conceived through IVF now account for about 1% of all live births. Its primary aim is to create at least one good quality embryo outside the body for transfer to the uterus, bypassing the tubes. Additional embryos may be frozen for future use. Success rates vary, but in the United Kingdom they are 28.2% per cycle started in the under-35 age group and 10% per cycle started in the 40–42-year-old age group.[4] IVF may be used to treat both female and male factor infertility as well as unexplained infertility.

In order to obtain several good quality embryos it is necessary to stimulate the ovaries to produce many eggs. There are many different protocols for superovulation. Most protocols involve using a gonadotrophin-releasing hormone (GnRH) agonist to 'downregulate' the pituitary gland. Once downregulation is achieved, gonadotrophins (either urinary FSH or recombinant FSH) are used to stimulate follicle production. Follicular development is tracked with serial ultrasound scans until at least three follicles of diameter greater or equal to 18 mm are seen. Subcutaneous human chorionic gonadotrophin (hCG) is administered and the oocytes are retrieved 34–38 hours post-hCG injection.

After retrieval, the oocytes are fertilized, cultured and then replaced. In cases of severe male factor infertility, such as azoospermia or when semen quality is very poor, ICSI may be required to achieve fertilization. Micromanipulators are used to inject a single sperm into the egg. Fertilization rates as high as standard IVF can be achieved in this way, even with extremely poor sperm.

Egg donation

Egg donation is rarely a first-line treatment, as ovulation induction will usually be attempted first. Oocyte donation may be appropriate after repeated failed attempts at IVF. In addition, it is used in cases of premature ovarian failure or conditions such as

Table 19.1 Currently used techniques for assisted reproduction
Ovulation induction
Intrauterine insemination
Donor insemination
In vitro fertilization (IVF)
IVF with intracytoplasmic sperm injection (ICSI)
Egg donation

Turner's syndrome in which women do not produce their own eggs. Donors are screened in a similar way to sperm donors.

Careful counselling is required before the use of donor gametes. It is important that the couple are aware that any child born using donated gametes has the right to identifiable information about their genetic donor when they reach 18 years of age.

Which surgical procedures might improve the chances of conception?

If tubal occlusion is diagnosed (or indeed the patient has been previously sterilized), tubal surgery is a possible option. There is debate about the value of tubal surgery and many clinicians would advocate IVF rather than tubal surgery as a first-line treatment. However, tubal surgery (apart from reversal of sterilization) may be funded by a healthcare provider when IVF is not, and so for many couples a chance of success with tubal surgery is the only option available to them. Cumulative pregnancy rates after surgery range between 25% and over 70%, depending on the type of procedure.[5,6] Success rates depend on the degree of tubal damage and are higher if the blockage is proximal rather than distal. Women undergoing tubal surgery must be warned of the significant risk of subsequent ectopic pregnancy.

In women who are known to have hydrosalpinges and tubal occlusion, laparoscopic salpingectomy should be offered prior to IVF. This has been shown to increase the live birth rate.[7] Women who are known to have minimal to mild endometriosis should be offered laparoscopy and ablation of the endometriosis. This has been shown to increase pregnancy and live birth rates in spontaneous conception.[8]

What irreversible factors would affect the outcome of assisted reproduction treatments (ART)?

Approximately seven million germ cells are found in fetal ovaries. These cells are lost at a rate of 30 to 40 per month throughout life including, for example, through pregnancy and contraceptive use. Only two million are left at birth and 300 000 by menarche.[9] The rate of depletion varies between individuals but after the age of 35 years, fertility declines rapidly. Increasing female age is the most significant factor in poor ART outcome.

The ability of the ovaries to respond to gonadotrophins with adequate follicular development is known as ovarian reserve. Ovarian reserve is not simply related to age, as women of the same age may have very different ovarian reserves. The measurement of day 2 to day 5 FSH is an indirect measurement of ovarian reserve.

Elevated FSH has been shown to be associated with poor pregnancy rates after assisted reproduction and high miscarriage rates, regardless of age.[10] Pregnancy rates decline significantly as FSH rises above 15 IU/l. Very few pregnancies have been reported when FSH levels exceed 25 IU/l.[11,12] However, there is no consensus regarding routine testing of ovarian reserve (see Case 18: Subfertility Investigations).

Recent Developments

Cumulative evidence from large cohort studies, multicentre studies, and meta-analyses suggests that assisted reproductive technologies are associated with an elevated risk of congenital malformations.[13] Theoretically, there are several factors in infertility treatments which could contribute to the development of congenital malformations. These include the exposure to gonadotrophin stimulation and the exposure to supra-physiological levels of E2; the altered physiological environment of implantation; the *in vitro* culture conditions at early stages of embryonic development; the artificial selection of sperm for fertilization and the sperm injection process in ICSI; and the process of embryo cryopreservation. However, it is also possible that the culprit is a factor or factors inherent to infertile patients. A review undertaken by Farhi and Fisch[13] confirmed the increased risk of congenital malformations in relation to *in vitro* fertilization even in singleton infants. There was no difference in the occurrence of major congenital malformations by either the laboratory procedures of sperm or embryos of varying complexity or by the specific medications used for ovarian stimulation or luteal support. Increased risk for congenital malformations was also found in infertile couples in relation to infertility treatment with ovulation induction with or without intrauterine insemination and even in spontaneous conception. They conclude that infertile couples have an inherent, *a priori* risk for congenital malformations in their offspring. The risk increases in direct relation to the severity of infertility treatment by which the pregnancy was obtained.

Conclusion

 It is becoming clear that there are other as yet unidentified factors, such as factors affecting implantation, which affect the outcome of ART. It is important that couples realize that, in some cases, even prolonged treatment may not result in pregnancy.[14]

Further Reading

1 Hughes E, Collins J, Vandekerckhove P. Clomiphene citrate for ovulation induction in women with oligo-amenorrhoea. *Cochrane Database Syst Rev* 2000; CD000056.

2 Fujii S, Fukui A, Fukushi Y, Kagiya A, Sato S, Saito Y. The effects of clomiphene citrate on normally ovulatory women. *Fertil Steril* 1997; **68**: 997–9.

3 National Institute for Health and Clinical Excellence. Fertility assessment and treatment for people with fertility problems. February 2004. www.nice.org.uk/guidance/CG11/guidance/pdf/English

4 The Human Fertility and Embryology Authority. www.hfea.gov.uk

5 Gomel V, McComb PF. Microsurgery for tubal infertility. *J Reprod Med* 2006; **51**: 177–84.

6 Sacks G, Trew G. Reconstruction, destruction and IVF: dilemmas in the art of tubal surgery. *BJOG* 2004; **111**: 1174–81.

7 Johnson NP, Mak W, Sowter MC. Surgical treatment for tubal disease in women due to undergo in vitro fertilisation. *Cochrane Database Syst Rev* 2001; CD002125.

8 Jacobson TZ, Barlow DH, Koninckx PR, Olive D, Farquhar C. Laparoscopic surgery for subfertilty associated with endometriosis. *Cochrane Database Syst Rev* 2002; CD001398.

9 Gosden RG. Follicular status at the menopause. *Hum Reprod* 1987; **2**: 617–21.

10 Levi AJ, Raynault MF, Bergh PA, Drews MR, Miller BT, Scott RT Jr. Reproductive outcomes in patients with diminished ovarian reserve. *Fertil Steril* 2001; **76**: 666–9.

11 Scott RT, Toner JP, Muasher SJ, Oehninger S, Robinson S, Rosenwaks Z. Follicle-stimulating hormone levels on cycle day 3 are predictive of in vitro fertilization outcome. *Fertil Steril* 1989; **51**: 651–4.

12 Maheshwari A, Fowler P, Bhattacharya S. Assessment of ovarian reserve—should we perform tests of ovarian reserve routinely? *Hum Reprod* 2006; **21**: 2729–35.

13 Farhi J, Fisch B. Risk of major congenital malformations associated with infertility and its treatment by extent of iatrogenic intervention. *Pediatr Endocrinol Rev* 2007; **4**: 352–7.

14 Covington SN, Hammer Burns L. *Infertility Counseling: A Comprehensive Handbook for Clinicians*, 2nd edn. Cambridge, NY, USA: Cambridge University Press, 2006.

PROBLEM

20 Optimizing Assisted Conception

Case History

A woman attends your clinic. She has been trying to conceive for six months. She is known to have polycystic ovary syndrome (PCOS) and has a body mass index (BMI) of 37 kg/m². She comes to see you because she feels that at 34 years of age, 'time is not on her side'. Her partner is 35 years old and is fit and well.

What general lifestyle advice would you give her?

What advice specific to her PCOS and weight would you give her?

What treatments may be appropriate for her?

Background

What general lifestyle advice would you give her?
Smoking

Women who smoke are known to have reduced fertility and therefore advice and information about smoking cessation programmes should be offered. Even passive smoking may be associated with delayed conception. The relationship between male smoking and fertility is unclear although it is associated with reduced semen parameters.

Alcohol and recreational drugs

It is known that excessive alcohol can damage the developing fetus. There is no strong evidence regarding alcohol intake pre-conception. However the United Kingdom Department of Health recommends women who are trying to conceive drink no more than one or two units of alcohol, once or twice a week.[1] Excessive alcohol is known to affect semen quality but its effect is reversible. Recreational drugs are known to affect fertility potential. Marijuana and cocaine can affect ovulatory function. Cocaine and anabolic steroids may also affect semen quality.

Medications

There is evidence that non-steroidal anti-inflammatory drugs (NSAIDs) inhibit ovulation.[2] Drugs including thyroxine, antidepressants, asthma medication and tranquillizers may also increase the risk of anovulatory infertility.[3]

Supplements

Folic acid supplementation does not increase chances of conception, but a dose of 400 μg daily pre-conception should be recommended to all women who are trying to conceive. This is because it has been shown to reduce the incidence of neural tube defects.

Vitamin supplements do not affect the chances of pregnancy but it should be remembered that women who are trying to conceive or who are pregnant should avoid high doses of vitamin A which is teratogenic.

In women with a normal haemoglobin level there is no evidence that iron supplementation is either beneficial or harmful. Advice regarding a balanced diet should be offered.

Exercise

General advice regarding exercise, especially during pregnancy, should be offered. Maternal benefits of exercise may be both physical and psychological.[4] Women who exercise in pregnancy may be less likely to develop some pregnancy complications such as swelling, varicosities and fatigue. Women who exercise more also experience less anxiety, stress and depression. Women with pregnancies complicated by medical conditions should consult their medical team for advice specific to their condition.

Rubella

Rubella infection during early pregnancy can result in significant congenital abnormalities. The routine use of the live attenuated rubella vaccine has significantly decreased the incidence of congenital rubella. However around 2% of subfertile women will be susceptible. Women who wish to conceive should therefore be screened to assess their immune status and the vaccine should be offered if they are susceptible. Pregnancy should be avoided for at least one month after vaccination because of the risk of teratogenicity.

What advice specific to her PCOS and weight would you give her?

A woman with PCOS is more likely to ovulate if she reduces her BMI to below 30 kg/m^2. If she finds weight loss difficult it may be appropriate to encourage her to join a supervised weight-reduction programme, as they have been shown to help reduce weight and in turn increase ovulation and conception rates.[5]

It is important that any woman who is overweight is made aware that if she does become pregnant, the risks to both her and her fetus are significant.[6] The operative delivery rate has been found to be increased with maternal obesity: 33.8% in the obese, 47.4% in the morbidly obese and 20.7% in women with a normal BMI.

Obese women have a significantly higher risk of pre-eclampsia than women with a normal BMI (13.5% versus 3.9%) as well as pregnancy-induced hypertension. In addition, they are more likely to develop venous thromboembolism. Obese women are 3.6 times more likely to develop gestational diabetes and in the long term are more likely to develop type 2 diabetes.

Perinatal mortality is higher in the obese population: 5.7 per 1000 births compared with 1.4 per 1000 of the population with a normal BMI. Ante-partum stillbirth is more than three times as likely in the morbidly obese population when compared to women with a normal BMI.[6]

Given these risks, women should be asked to reduce their weight to a BMI below 35 kg/m² before treatment for subfertility is initiated.[7]

What treatments may be appropriate for her?

In women who are not ovulating, clomifene is usually the first line of treatment. About 70% of anovulatory women will ovulate in response to clomifene although only 40%–50% will conceive.[8] Ultrasound monitoring of the ovaries should be performed in the first cycle (Figure 20.1).

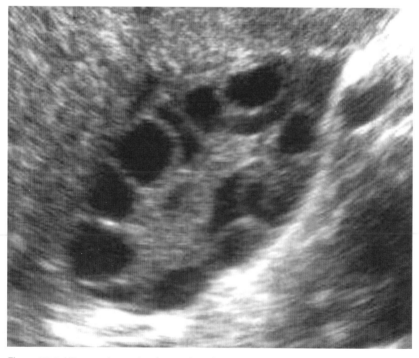

Figure 20.1 Ultrasound scan showing a polycystic ovary.

Another method of ovulation induction in women with PCOS is laparoscopic ovarian drilling. This is as effective as using gonadotrophins to induce ovulation in women with PCOS but does not carry the same risk of multiple pregnancy.[9] Its disadvantage is the significant risk associated with laparoscopy in women who are often overweight. However, if there is a clinical reason to perform laparoscopy, such as suspected pelvic pathology (for example, tubal disease or endometriosis), ovarian drilling may be performed at the same time.

Recent Developments

The use of metformin has attracted attention but the results are contradictory. A meta-analysis of 13 randomized trials comparing metformin with placebo, or metformin plus clomifene with clomifene alone, in women with PCOS concluded that metformin increased the ovulation rate by a factor of approximately four.[10] However, pregnancy rates did not differ significantly between the metformin groups and the placebo groups, although the pregnancy rates for metformin plus clomifene were significantly higher than for clomifene alone.[10] An Italian trial of 100 infertile, non-obese women with PCOS showed similar rates of ovulation with either metformin or clomifene, although the pregnancy rate in the metformin group was twice that in the clomifene group.[11] However, in a randomized trial that compared clomifene plus metformin with clomifene plus placebo in 225 infertile Dutch women with PCOS (mean BMI 28 kg/m^2), the addition of metformin did not significantly improve rates of either ovulation or pregnancy.[12] Clomifene citrate plus placebo, extended-release metformin plus placebo, or a combination of metformin and clomifene for up to six months has been evaluated in a United States randomized controlled trial.[13] The live birth rate was 22.5% in the clomifene group, 7.2% in the metformin group and 26.8% in the combination therapy group. However, the conception rate among subjects who ovulated was significantly lower in the metformin group (21.7%) than in either the clomifene group (39.5%) or the combination therapy group (46.0%). Thus, while women with PCOS are at increased risk for the metabolic syndrome and metformin may well be important in treating these metabolic disturbances, its metabolic benefits do not translate into live birth rates that are as high as those with clomifene.[14]

Conclusion

The issue of obesity in pregnancy has come to the fore with the current obesity epidemic.
It is essential for women to normalize their weight prior to pregnancy. This will increase her chances of conception, reduce pregnancy complications and perinatal mortality.

Further Reading

1 Mueller BA, Daling JR, Weiss NS, Moore DE. Recreational drug use and the risk of primary infertility. *Epidemiology* 1990; 1: 195–200.

2 Stone S, Khamashta MA, Nelson-Piercy C. Nonsteroidal anti-inflammatory drugs and reversible female infertility: is there a link? *Drug Saf* 2002; **25**: 545–51.

3 Poppe K, Velkeniers B, Glinoer D. Thyroid disease and female reproduction. *Clin Endocrinol (Oxf)* 2007; **66**: 309–21.

4 Weissgerber TL, Wolfe LA, Davies GA, Mottola MF. Exercise in the prevention and treatment of maternal-fetal disease: a review of the literature. *Appl Physiol Nutr Metab* 2006; **31**: 661–74.

5 Crosignani PG, Colombo M, Vegetti W, Somigliana E, Gessati A, Ragni G. Overweight and obese anovulatory patients with polycystic ovaries: parallel improvements in anthropometric indices, ovarian physiology and fertility rate induced by diet. *Hum Reprod* 2003; **18**: 1928–32.

6 Yu CK, Teoh TG, Robinson S. Obesity in pregnancy. *BJOG* 2006; **113**: 1117–25.

7 Gillett WR, Putt T, Farquhar CM. Prioritising for fertility treatments—the effect of excluding women with a high body mass index. *BJOG* 2006; **113**: 1218–21.

8 Palomba S, Orio F, Zullo F. Ovulation induction in women with polycystic ovary syndrome. *Fertil Steril* 2006; **86** (Suppl 1): S26–7.

9 Farquhar C, Vandekerckhove P, Lilford R. Laparoscopic "drilling" by diathermy or laser for ovulation induction in anovulatory polycystic ovarian syndrome. *Cochrane Database Syst Rev* 2001; CD001122.

10 Lord JM, Flight IHK, Norman RJ. Metformin in polycystic ovary syndrome: systematic review and meta-analysis. *BMJ* 2003; **327**: 951–3.

11 Palomba S, Orio F Jr, Falbo A, Manguso F, Russo T, Cascella T, Tolino A, Carmina E, Colao A, Zullo F. Prospective parallel randomized, double-blind, double-dummy controlled clinical trial comparing clomiphene citrate and metformin as the first-line treatment for ovulation induction in nonobese anovulatory women with polycystic ovary syndrome. *J Clin Endocrinol Metab* 2005; **90**: 4068–74.

12 Moll EBP, Bossuyt PM, Korevaar JC, Lambalk CB, van der Veen F. Effect of clomifene citrate plus metformin and clomifene citrate plus placebo on induction of ovulation in women with newly diagnosed polycystic ovary syndrome: randomized double blind clinical trial. *BMJ* 2006; **332**: 1485.

13 Legro RS, Barnhart HX, Schlaff WD, Carr BR, Diamond MP, Carson SA, Steinkampf MP, Coutifaris C, McGovern PG, Cataldo NA, Gosman GG, Nestler JE, Giudice LC, Leppert PC, Myers ER; Cooperative Multicenter Reproductive Medicine Network. Clomiphene, metformin, or both for infertility in the polycystic ovary syndrome. *N Engl J Med* 2007; **356**: 551–66.

14 Carmina E. Metabolic syndrome in polycystic ovary syndrome. *Minerva Ginecol* 2006; **58**: 109–14.

21 Egg Cryopreservation

Case History

A 32-year-old nulliparous woman comes to your clinic having been diagnosed with breast cancer. She has recently had surgery but has been told that she requires chemotherapy. She has read that it is possible to freeze eggs so that once her chemotherapy is over she may still have the chance of having children who are genetically her own.

How would you advise her as to the success rates of oocyte cryopreservation?

What are the risks of ovulation induction in a woman with breast cancer?

What alternatives to oocyte cryopreservation are available to her?

Background

Approximately 15% of breast cancers occur before the age of 45 years. Treatment with adjuvant chemotherapy is well recognized as a cause of infertility.[1] The younger the woman and the greater her ovarian reserve, the less likely she is to become menopausal as a consequence of chemotherapy. However, even young women are likely to become menopausal earlier than they otherwise would have done, as a consequence of chemotherapy. Given the increasing numbers of women who delay childbirth, there are significant numbers of women who develop breast cancer and have to face the prospect of infertility.[2] It has been found that concerns regarding fertility influenced the treatment decisions of almost a third of young women with breast cancer.[3]

How would you advise her as to the success rates of oocyte cryopreservation?

It has been possible for many years to cryopreserve sperm in order to preserve fertility in men who need treatment with chemotherapy or radiotherapy which is likely to compromise their fertility. Frozen sperm does not fertilize oocytes as effectively as fresh sperm and intracytoplasmic sperm injection (ICSI) is usually required.

In recent years there has been increasing research attempting to successfully preserve human oocytes. This has been done either to preserve future fertility for women undergoing cancer treatment or to protect against the decreased fertility of the ageing ovary in women wishing to have children later in life. The first pregnancy resulting from oocyte cryopreservation was reported in 1986.[4]

As this is a relatively new technique, there is a lack of good data on oocyte cryopreservation and thus it remains difficult to counsel women. A meta-analysis of reported oocyte cryopreservation programmes showed a live birth rate per oocyte thawed of 1.9%–2.0%. If the oocyte survived the freeze–thaw and ICSI was performed, the live birth rate was 3.4%. If embryo transfer took place, the live birth rate was 21.6%.[5]

The technology surrounding oocyte cryopreservation continues to develop rapidly and survival rates of cryopreserved oocytes will no doubt continue to improve. For women with cancer who wish to preserve fertility but do not want to proceed to embryo cryopreservation, egg cryopreservation may be an acceptable option. Conversely, in women who wish oocyte preservation only to delay childbearing, it cannot be stressed too strongly that the success rates are low and meanwhile their natural fertility is diminishing.

What are the risks of ovulation induction in a woman with breast cancer?

Conventional protocols for ovulation induction will usually result in a 10–15-fold increase in the normal physiological oestradiol level. The effects of such high levels of oestrogen on what are often oestrogen-dependent tumours are unknown. Therefore, women with breast cancer wishing to undergo ovulation induction must be carefully counselled about the potential and theoretical risks.

There is commonly a period of six weeks between primary surgery and the start of chemotherapy. Ovulation induction may take place during this interval. It is important to note that there must be an adequate recovery time between egg collection and the commencement of chemotherapy. This is because ovulation induction and egg collection carry significant risks (Table 21.1) such as ovarian hyperstimulation syndrome and pelvic infection. If chemotherapy is commenced prior to the identification of a complication such as infection, the result could be catastrophic for the woman.

Women with breast cancer who have embryos or eggs frozen are usually advised to delay conception for at least two years after treatment. This allows time to differentiate women with a better prognosis from those who have aggressive disease. Younger women are known to often have more aggressive disease. Therefore women under the age of 33 years may be well advised to delay pregnancy for three years.[6] However, a shorter delay has been suggested.[7]

The psychological consequences of fertility treatment under these circumstances must not be underestimated. Couples may feel that the creation of frozen embryos can only be positive. However, several years down the line if the tumour recurs or the relationship

Table 21.1 Risks of assisted reproduction	
Technique	Risks
Ovulation induction	Ovarian hyperstimulation syndrome
	Multiple pregnancy
Egg collection	Infection
	Damage to bladder/bowel
Embryo transfer	Ectopic pregnancy
Multiple pregnancy	Prematurity
	Ante-partum haemorrhage/post-partum haemorrhage
	Pre-eclampsia

ends, couples may be faced with difficult dilemmas such as how to use or dispose of the embryos.

What alternatives to oocyte cryopreservation are available to her?

If the woman has a partner, or would consider the use of donor sperm, *in vitro* fertilization and cryopreservation of embryos, rather than oocytes, should be considered to be the first-line management. The live birth rate following embryo cryopreservation and subsequent transfer now approaches the success rates of fresh cycles in many units.[8] There will be, however, some women who for religious or personal reasons will not agree to embryo cryopreservation or the use of donor sperm.

It is essential that women understand the clear differences between these two procedures. Oocyte cryopreservation remains experimental whilst embryo cryopreservation is now a standard part of every fertility centre's practice, with often excellent pregnancy rates achieved.[9]

In patients who have a cancer which requires them to have pelvic irradiation, transposition of the ovaries can be performed to remove the ovaries from a site vulnerable to irradiation.

Other possibilities, such as the use of donor oocytes or adoption, should be discussed with patients contemplating ovulation induction and the cryopreservation of embryos or oocytes. For some, surrogacy may be a possibility.

Recent Developments

1 Experimental work is underway in both cryopreservation of ovarian tissue and transplantation of ovarian tissue in order to preserve fertility in women undergoing treatment for cancer. As yet, few live births have been achieved using these methods.[9]

2 Data on birth outcome and offspring health after breast cancer are limited.[10] A population study of all 2 870 932 singleton births registered in the Swedish Medical Birth Registry during 1973–2002 identified 331 first births following breast cancer surgery. The large majority of births from women previously treated for breast cancer had no adverse events. However, births by women exposed to breast cancer were associated with an increased risk of delivery complications (odds ratio [OR] 1.5; 95% confidence interval [CI] 1.2–1.9), Caesarean section (OR 1.3; 95% CI 1.0–1.7), very preterm birth (<32 wk) (OR 3.2; 95% CI 1.7–6.0), and low birth weight (<1500 g) (OR 2.9; 95% CI 1.4–5.8). A tendency towards an increased risk of malformations among the infants was seen especially in the later time period (1988–2002) (OR 2.1; 95% CI 1.2–3.7). Thus, pregnancies in previously treated breast cancer patients could be regarded as higher risk pregnancies.

Conclusion

The decision for this patient is difficult. She must be made aware of the risks of ovulation induction and the uncertainties regarding recurrence on a young family.

Further Reading

1 Goodwin PJ, Ennis M, Pritchard KI, Trudeau M, Hood N. Risk of menopause during the first year after breast cancer diagnosis. *J Clin Oncol* 1999; **17**: 2365–70.

2 Sonmezer M, Oktay K. Fertility preservation in young women undergoing breast cancer therapy. *Oncologist* 2006; **11**: 422–34.

3 Partridge AH, Gelber S, Peppercorn J, Sampson E, Knudsen K, Laufer M, Rosenberg R, Przypyszny M, Rein A, Winer EP. Web-based survey of fertility issues in young women with breast cancer. *J Clin Oncol* 2004; **22**: 4174–83.

4 Chen C. Pregnancy after human oocyte cryopreservation. *Lancet* 1986; **1**: 884–6.

5 Oktay K, Cil AP, Bang H. Efficiency of oocyte cryopreservation: a meta analysis. *Fertil Steril* 2006; **86**: 70–80.

6 Veeck LL, Bodine R, Clarke RN, Berrios R, Libraro J, Moschini RM, Zaninovic N, Rosenwaks Z. High pregnancy rates can be achieved after freezing and thawing human blastocysts. *Fertil Steril* 2004; **82**: 1418–27.

7 Ives A, Saunders C, Bulsara M, Semmens J. Pregnancy after breast cancer: population based study. *BMJ* 2007; **334**: 194.

8 Oktay K, Buyuk E, Davis OK, Veeck L, Rosenwaks Z. A prospective comparison of tamoxifen alone and tamoxifen-FSH combined protocol for IVF and fertility preservation in breast cancer patients. *Fertil Steril* 2003; **80** (Suppl 3): 63–4.

9 Donnez J, Martinez-Madrid B, Jadoul P, Van Langendonckt A, Demylle D, Dolmans MM. Ovarian tissue cryopreservation and transplantation: a review. *Hum Reprod Update* 2006; **12**: 519–35.

10 Dalberg K, Eriksson J, Holmberg L. Birth outcome in women with previously treated breast cancer – a population-based cohort study from Sweden. *PLoS Med* 2006; **3**: e336.

22 Recurrent Miscarriage

Case History

A 29-year-old woman and her 30-year-old partner have been trying to conceive for two years and during that time she has had three miscarriages, all occurring between seven and nine weeks. She is otherwise fit and well but her mother suffered a pulmonary embolus during pregnancy.

What further tests would you arrange?

What causes of recurrent miscarriage should be considered?

What is the outlook for future pregnancies?

Background

Recurrent miscarriage is defined as three miscarriages occurring consecutively. Miscarriage is common, affecting about one in six pregnancies.[1] One might expect, therefore, that a third consecutive miscarriage might occur by chance in about 1 in 200 pregnancies. In fact, recurrent miscarriage affects about 1% of couples.

What further tests would you arrange?

Generally, couples are advised not to have further investigations until they have suffered three losses.[2] This is because investigations may reveal abnormal results which may have no clinical significance but which are subsequently linked to the miscarriage. Inappropriate and potentially dangerous treatment may consequently be initiated. For the majority of women suffering a miscarriage, even a repeated miscarriage, it would have been caused by a sporadic fetal lethal chromosomal or structural abnormality. The loss of an established pregnancy with a fetal heart after ten weeks is relatively unusual and some argue that investigation should be initiated after one such loss. Table 22.1 outlines the tests that are recommended for the investigation of recurrent miscarriage.

What causes of recurrent miscarriage should be considered?

Chromosomal analysis for both male and female

Balanced translocations (Figure 22.1) occur in one partner in 3%–5% of couples in the recurrent miscarriage population. The individual concerned has no health problems, but his or her gametes will have too little or too much genetic material and will repeatedly form abnormal embryos. Couples should be referred to a geneticist for further advice.

Table 221   Investigation of recurrent miscarriage
● Blood karyotype for male and female
● Thrombophilia screen
● Antiphospholipid antibodies
● Anticardiolipin
● Lupus anticoagulant

● Hormone profile
   – Follicle-stimulating hormone, luteinizing hormone, testosterone
   – Glucose or thyroid function test if symptomatic

● Transvaginal ultrasound scan for uterine anomaly

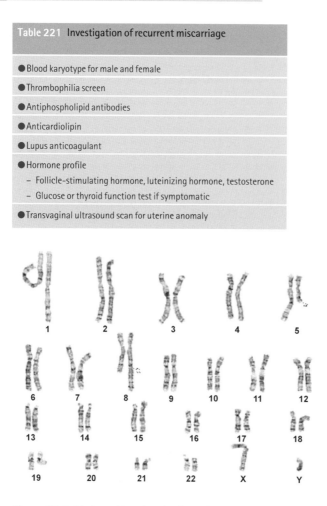

Figure 22.1 A balanced translocation from chromosome 5 to chromosome 8.

Pre-implantation genetic diagnosis may be a possibility but should be balanced against the reduced fertility associated with *in vitro* fertilization in a healthy fertile couple.

Antiphospholipid syndrome

The presence of anticardiolipin antibodies and lupus anticoagulant are associated with recurrent miscarriage.[3,4] These antibodies occur in the population at a rate of approximately 2%, but are present in 15% of women with recurrent miscarriage. Two samples, taken at least six weeks apart, showing moderate or high levels of immunoglobulin (Ig) G and/or IgM should be positive before a diagnosis is made. The syndrome requires the presence of antibodies in association with one of the following clinical events:

● vascular thrombosis

● three consecutive early pregnancy losses

- one established pregnancy (i.e. fetal heart seen) after ten weeks or
- delivery before 34 weeks associated with severe pre-eclampsia

The likely mechanism of pregnancy loss may involve defective trophoblast implantation in the initial stages of pregnancy and/or later thrombosis within the placenta. Treatments involving heparin and aspirin have been successful in reducing pregnancy loss but have significant side effects, in particular the development of osteopenia during pregnancy.[4] Although the live birth rate may be improved from 10% to 70% with treatment, the pregnancies remain high risk.

Thrombophilia screen

Some inherited forms of clotting abnormality may be associated with miscarriage. Deficiencies in protein C (most commonly due to the Factor V Leiden mutation), protein S and antithrombin III have been identified as possible relevant defects.[5] However, the value of treatment of these inherited defects remains uncertain. Heparin, with and without aspirin, has been studied but results have not shown benefit. Further studies are needed and patients may wish to take part in such research.[6]

Metabolic abnormalities

Poorly controlled diabetes is associated with an increased rate of miscarriage but this would be an unusual presentation of diabetes. Similarly, thyroid abnormalities are common and should be treated prior to pregnancy but are unlikely to present with recurrent miscarriage. Tests screening for thyroid abnormalities and diabetes should not be done in asymptomatic women.

Follicle-stimulating hormone (FSH) and luteinizing hormone (LH) should be checked on day 2–5 of the cycle. An unusually high level of FSH might point towards poor ovarian reserve and perhaps poorer quality eggs, which would account for an increased rate of miscarriage. A high LH/FSH ratio might point towards polycystic ovaries and may be associated with a high testosterone level. With ultrasound examination, a diagnosis of polycystic ovaries can be made and this is more common among the recurrent miscarriage population. However, if spontaneous conception occurs, women with polycystic ovaries on ultrasound scan are not more likely than other women to suffer a miscarriage. Treatments to suppress the LH level in women with polycystic ovaries do not improve the live birth rate, but there is some evidence to suggest that metformin may reduce the rate of miscarriage in women with polycystic ovary syndrome.[7]

Progesterone supplementation does not reduce the risk of miscarriage in women who have suffered recurrent pregnancy loss. The falling progesterone levels seen in this situation probably reflect the poor prognosis of the pregnancy.

Uterine anomalies

Second trimester abnormalities are certainly associated with uterine abnormalities such as uterine septum and incompetent cervix. In the first trimester this is harder to demonstrate but it is appropriate to investigate the possibility of uterine abnormality, which is usually done initially using a transvaginal ultrasound scan (TVS). Further imaging using magnetic resonance imaging (MRI) or hysterosalpingography may be helpful. It is not at all clear that treating any detected uterine abnormality will improve the live birth rate and may create additional reproductive complications such as infertility and scar rupture.[8]

Alloimmune conditions

Despite widespread interest in these conditions, there is no evidence that any of the available tests identify pathological states nor that recommended treatments improve outcome.[9,10]

What is the outlook for future pregnancies?

For many couples, the test results will all be normal, and three-quarters of them will go on to carry a normal pregnancy to term. In this situation the aim of treatment is to offer any reassurance that may be helpful, such as access to regular scanning.

Recent Developments

Oxidative stress-induced damage has been hypothesized to play a role in idiopathic recurrent pregnancy loss.[11] Some studies implicate systemic and placental oxidative stress in the pathophysiology of abortion and recurrent pregnancy loss. Oxidant-induced endothelial damage, impaired placental vascularization and immune malfunction have all been proposed to play a role. Oxidative stress-induced modification of phospholipids has been linked to the formation of antiphospholipid antibodies in the antiphospholipid syndrome.

Conclusion

The management of recurrent miscarriage is an extremely emotional area and couples will clutch at any treatment to achieve success. Many treatments have been suggested which were subsequently shown to be unhelpful or dangerous. It is suggested, therefore, that treatment should not be used unless it has been shown to be effective. It may be best to refer such patients to specialist clinics.

Further Reading

1 Duckitt K, Qureshi A. Recurrent miscarriage. *Clin Evid* 2006; **15**: 1986–95.

2 Royal College of Obstetricians and Gynaecologists (RCOG). *The Investigation and Treatment of Couples with Recurrent Miscarriage*. Green-top Guideline No. 17. London: RCOG Press, 2003.

3 Rai R, Regan L. Recurrent miscarriage. *Lancet* 2006; **368**: 601–11.

4 Empson M, Lassere M, Craig J, Scott J. Prevention of recurrent miscarriage for women with antiphospholipid antibody or lupus anticoagulant. *The Cochrane Library*, Issue 3. Chichester: John Wiley & Sons, 2006.

5 Carp HJ. Thrombophilia and recurrent pregnancy loss. *Obstet Gynecol Clin North Am* 2006; **33**: 429–42.

6 Di Nisio M, Peters LW, Middeldorp S. Anticoagulants for the treatment of recurrent pregnancy loss in women without antiphospholipid syndrome. *The Cochrane Library*, Issue 3. Chichester: John Wiley & Sons, 2006.

7 Homburg R. Pregnancy complications in PCOS. *Best Pract Res Clin Endocrinol Metab* 2006; **20**: 281–92.

8 Devi Wold AS, Pham N, Arici A. Anatomic factors in recurrent pregnancy loss. *Semin Reprod Med* 2006; **24**: 25–32.

9 Porter TF, LaCoursiere Y, Scott JR. Immunotherapy for recurrent miscarriage. *The Cochrane Library*, Issue 3. Chichester: John Wiley & Sons, 2006.

10 Royal College of Obstetricians and Gynaecologists. *Immunological Testing and Interventions for Reproductive Failure.* Scientific Advisory Committee Opinion Paper No. 5. London: RCOG Press, 2003.

11 Gupta S, Agarwal A, Banerjee J, Alvarez JG. The role of oxidative stress in spontaneous abortion and recurrent pregnancy loss: a systematic review. *Obstet Gynecol Surv* 2007; **62**: 335–47.

PROBLEM

23 Unplanned Pregnancy

Case History

A 21-year-old woman requests a pregnancy test. She normally has regular periods but this month her period is late and she has noticed some breast tenderness and nausea. She is very clear that she would not wish to continue with a pregnancy under any circumstances. An early morning sample of urine tested in the clinic confirms a positive pregnancy test.

What are the important questions to ask when taking a history?

What are the options for termination of pregnancy?

What are the important aspects of follow-up?

Background

Induced abortion or termination of pregnancy (TOP) is a very common gynaecological procedure. In the United States in 2003, 848 163 legal induced abortions were reported to the Centers for Disease Control and Prevention.[1] According to the World Health Organization, in countries where induced abortion is permitted by law, which have total fertility rates of about 2 or less and high prevalence rates of contraceptive use, the annual rate of induced abortion is 1 to 2 abortions per 100 women of reproductive age.[2] In countries with similar fertility rates but much lower prevalence of contraceptive use, the annual rate of induced abortion is higher and can be estimated to be up to 10 or more per 100 women annually. In countries where abortion is permitted by law, the large majority of abortions (typically >90%) take place before the end of the 12th week of pregnancy. Legislation about abortion varies throughout the world, may vary within different states of an individual country and may be illegal in some countries.[1, 3, 4] The upper time limit for legal induced abortion also varies. In Europe it ranges from 12–28 weeks. The statutory grounds for TOP in England are detailed in Table 23.1. The legal time limit for abortion is 24 weeks for clauses C and D. However, abortions after 24 weeks are allowed if there is grave risk to the life of the woman, evidence of severe fetal abnormality, or risk of grave physical and mental injury to the woman (clauses A, B and E).

Table 23.1 Statutory grounds for termination of pregnancy in England
A The continuance of the pregnancy would involve risk to the life of the pregnant woman greater than if the pregnancy were terminated
B The termination is necessary to prevent grave permanent injury to the physical or mental health of the pregnant woman
C The pregnancy has NOT exceeded its 24th week and that the continuance of the pregnancy would involve risk, greater than if the pregnancy were terminated, of injury to the physical or mental health of the pregnant woman
D The pregnancy has NOT exceeded its 24th week and that the continuance of the pregnancy would involve risk, greater than if the pregnancy were terminated, of injury to the physical or mental health of any existing child(ren) of the family of the pregnant woman
E There is a substantial risk that if the child were born it would suffer from such physical or mental abnormalities as to be seriously handicapped

What are the important questions to ask when taking a history?

When seen in the clinic, the patient should be made to feel at ease and given time to discuss and consider her options.[5] If possible, she should be advised to discuss with her partner, family or friends and return to the clinic having had time to arrive at a decision.

If the woman feels sure that she does not wish to continue with the pregnancy, there are several important points to consider when taking a history. The date of her last menstrual period, and whether it was normal, is essential to ascertain the likely gestation. Menstrual cycle length needs to be noted. It is important to establish whether any method of contraception has been used, as often women on the combined oral contraceptive (COC) pill may regard a withdrawal bleed as a period. A general medical and surgical history should be taken, as well as details of any current medication and drug allergies. Details of any previous pregnancies, and in particular ectopic pregnancy, should be recorded. A sexual history is important to assess the risk of sexually transmitted infection, and details of her last smear test should be obtained. An ultrasound scan needs to be undertaken if there is uncertainty about the date of the last menstrual period, uterine size on pelvic examination is not compatible with dates or she has risk factors for an ectopic pregnancy. Tests for chlamydia infection and other sexually transmitted diseases need to be undertaken according to local protocols (see Case 35: Sexually Transmitted Infections).

What are the options for termination of pregnancy?

The method of TOP available depends on the gestation of the pregnancy and the woman's choice.[5-7] The procedures offered also vary from one centre to another.

Surgical methods

Below seven weeks
Conventional suction termination should be avoided at gestations below seven weeks. Early surgical abortion using a rigorous protocol (which includes magnification of aspirated material and indications for serum β human chorionic gonadotrophin follow-up) may be used at gestations below seven weeks, although data suggest that the failure rate is higher than for medical abortion.

Thus, for women presenting at less than seven weeks of gestation, an alternative recommended technique should be chosen or the procedure deferred if possible.

At 7–15 weeks
Conventional suction termination is an appropriate method at gestations of 7–15 weeks, although, in some settings, the skills and experience of practitioners may make medical abortion more appropriate at gestations above twelve weeks.[8]

Above 15 weeks
For gestations above 15 weeks, surgical abortion by dilatation and evacuation, preceded by cervical preparation, is safe and effective when undertaken by specialist practitioners with access to the necessary instruments and who have a sufficiently large case load to maintain their skills.

Medical methods

Medical abortion using mifepristone plus prostaglandin is the most effective method of abortion at gestations of less than seven weeks and continues to be an appropriate method for women in the 7–9 week gestation band.

According to the Royal College of Obstetricians and Gynaecologists Guideline, medical abortion using the regimen below is a safe, effective and acceptable alternative to surgical abortion for women between 9 and 13 weeks of gestation.[5]

For mid-trimester abortion (13–24 weeks of gestation), medical abortion with mifepristone followed by prostaglandin is an appropriate method and has been shown to be safe and effective. Feticide may be considered in more advanced gestations.

- **Mifepristone (RU 486)** – is an antiprogesterone which binds to progesterone receptors in the uterus and other target organs, causes uterine contractions and bleeding from the placental bed and sensitizes the uterus to prostaglandins.

- **Misoprostol** – is a prostaglandin E1 analogue. It stimulates uterine contractions and is used in medical termination. It may also be useful for cervical preparation before surgical termination. Its use in TOP is off licence.

- **Gemeprost** – is a prostaglandin E1 analogue. It is licensed for softening and dilatation of the cervix before surgical termination in the first trimester, and for therapeutic TOP during the second trimester of pregnancy.

Blood tests should be taken for haemoglobin, blood group and Rhesus status and testing for haemaglobinopathies as indicated. Rhesus-negative women should receive anti-D immunoglobulin within 72 hours of TOP whether by surgical or medical methods.[5]

What are the important aspects of follow-up?

The purposes of follow-up after TOP are, firstly, to confirm successful abortion, and to identify possible complications from the procedure, to ensure adequate future contraception and to explore the psychological impact on the woman. Follow-up is generally offered within two weeks of the procedure.[9]

Complications of TOP include: haemorrhage (1 in 1000 overall; greater risk with later gestations); infection (up to 10% of cases and reduced by screening and prophylactic antibiotics); uterine perforation (1–4 in 1000); cervical trauma at the time of surgical abortion (no greater than 1 in 100); and failure (2.3 in 1000 surgical and 1–14 in 1000 medical, depending on the regimen used and the experience of the centre).[5] Induced abortion is not associated with an increased risk of breast cancer.[2,5] There are no proven associations between induced abortion and subsequent ectopic pregnancy, placenta praevia or infertility. With regard to psychological sequelae, the evidence is uncertain and may reflect underlying problems before the termination.

Abortion is usually confirmed through identifying the products of conception; however, a transvaginal ultrasound scan (TVS) of the uterus may be required.[9] The patient should be questioned regarding continued bleeding or pelvic pain. Routine chlamydia screening and use of prophylactic antibiotics is common practice, and follow-up of those testing positive for chlamydia infection is essential, including contact tracing.

Discussion regarding future contraception should ideally have taken place at the initial consultation and decisions made in advance, in case of non-attendance for follow-up. Women who receive specialist advice in advance are more likely to leave hospital with contraception and this is more likely to be a long-acting method.[9] Contraception administered at the time of surgical TOP has been found to be practical and effective, and most methods can be safely used following medical TOP, either initiated on the day of misoprostol administration (oral pills, condoms, injectable methods) or following the next menstrual cycle (intrauterine device or sterilization).[10]

Recent Developments

Despite guidelines and fact sheets stating that induced abortion does not increase the risk of breast cancer,[2,5] this can be an area of concern. The association between induced and spontaneous abortion and the incidence of breast cancer was studied in a prospective cohort of young women, the Nurses' Health Study II.[11] The study included 105 716 women 29 to 46 years old at the start of follow-up in 1993. During 973 437 person-years of follow-up between 1993 and 2003, 1458 newly diagnosed cases of invasive breast cancer were ascertained. A total of 16 118 participants (15%) reported a history of induced abortion, and 21 753 (21%) reported a history of spontaneous abortions. The hazard ratio for breast cancer among women who had one or more induced abortions was 1.01 (95% confidence interval [CI] 0.88–1.17) after adjustment for established breast cancer risk factors; among women with one or more spontaneous abortions, the covariate-adjusted hazard ratio was 0.89 (95% CI, 0.78–1.01). The relation between induced abortion and the incidence of breast cancer did not differ materially by number of abortions (P for trend = 0.98), age at abortion (P for trend = 0.68), parity (P for interaction = 0.54), or timing of abortion with respect to a full-term pregnancy (P for interaction = 0.10). This large study found that neither induced nor spontaneous abortion were associated with the incidence of breast cancer.

Conclusion

This patient is very clear that she wants an abortion and that she could not cope with a pregnancy at this stage of her life. She is found to be seven weeks pregnant and elects to have an early medical termination. Appropriate counselling should be offered, if available, for those having difficulty coming to terms with the procedure.

Further Reading

1 Strauss LT, Gamble SB, Parker WY, Cook DA, Zane SB, Hamdan S; Centers for Disease Control and Prevention. Abortion surveillance – United States, 2003. *MMWR Surveill Summ* 2006; **55**: 1–32.

2 World Health Organization. Induced abortion does not increase breast cancer risk. Fact sheet No. 240, June 2000. www.who.int/mediacentre/factsheets/fs240/en/ (accessed 19 09 07)

3 Bird S. Abortion and the law in Australia. *Aust Fam Physician* 2006; **35**: 905–6.

4 Pinter B, Aubeny E, Bartfai G, Loeber O, Ozalp S, Webb A. Accessibility and availability of abortion in six European countries. *Eur J Contracept Reprod Health Care* 2005; **10**: 51–8.

5 Royal College of Obstetricians and Gynaecologists (RCOG). *The Care of Women Requesting Induced Abortion.* Evidence-based Clinical Guideline No. 7. London: RCOG Press, 2004.

6 World Health Organization (WHO). *Safe abortion – technical and policy guidance for health systems.* Geneva: WHO Press, 2003.

7 Hamoda H, Flett GMM. Medical termination of pregnancy in the early first trimester. *J Fam Plann Reprod Health Care* 2005; **31**: 10–14.

8 Child TJ, Thomas J, Rees M, MacKenzie IZ. Morbidity of first trimester aspiration termination and the seniority of the surgeon. *Hum Reprod* 2001; **16**: 875–8.

9 Schunmann C, Glasier A. Specialist contraceptive counselling and provision after termination of pregnancy improves uptake of long-acting methods but does not prevent repeat abortion: a randomized trial. *Hum Reprod* 2006; **21**: 2296–303.

10 Mittal S. Contraception after medical abortion. *Contraception* 2006; **74**: 56–60.

11 Michels KB, Xue F, Colditz GA, Willett WC. Induced and spontaneous abortion and incidence of breast cancer among young women: a prospective cohort study. *Arch Intern Med* 2007; **167**: 814–20.

24 Preventing Teenage Pregnancy

Case History

A 14-year-old girl attends the clinic to discuss contraception. Her boyfriend is 17 years old and they have not yet had sex. She appears quite embarrassed and asks whether it would be a good idea for her to start the pill. She is very clear that she does not wish her parents to know about the consultation.

How would you approach the consultation?

How would you advise about sexually transmitted infections (STIs)?

What contraceptive methods would you advise?

Background

Despite a general trend towards later childbearing, teenage pregnancy remains a serious problem.[1] The incidence of teenage pregnancy varies widely throughout the world (Figure 24.1). In Europe the highest rate is in the United Kingdom and the lowest in the Netherlands and Switzerland.

Throughout most of western Europe, teenage birth rates fell during the 1970s, 1980s, and 1990s, but in the UK rates have remained high. However, for some young women, particularly from certain ethnic or social groups, teenage pregnancy can be a positive life choice. On the other hand, for many other young women, the costs of teenage pregnancy can be very high, particularly when linked with poverty. These risks include poorer outcomes for the children of teenage mothers as well as for the mothers themselves. Infant mortality among babies of teenage mothers is about 60% higher than among the babies of older mothers. Prevention of unwanted teenage pregnancies is a high priority in many countries and various strategies are used. High-quality evidence shows that health promotion behavioural programmes, using peer educators of a similar age, reduce the prevalence of sexual activity at age 16 years.[2,3] Although programmes that promote abstinence have a logical appeal, no high-quality studies have shown the effectiveness of such approaches.

How would you approach the consultation?

Young people often find it difficult to seek advice regarding sexual health for a number of reasons. Embarrassment, concerns about confidentiality and peer pressure can all affect the consultation. It is vitally important to try to ensure that the young person feels at ease

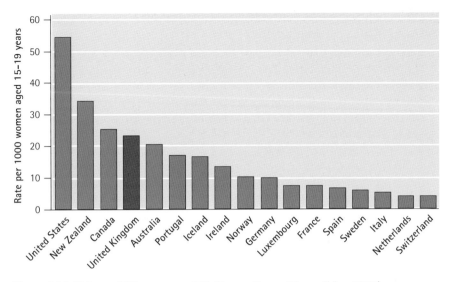

Figure 24.1 Births per 1000 women aged 15–19 years. *Source*: Tripp and Viner 1998.[1]

and to approach the consultation sensitively and in a non-judgemental manner. Instructions should be clear and concise and backed up with appropriate reading material, and if possible the patient should be seen alone if attending with a partner.

In this case, the patient is 14 years old and there may be child protection issues. The law varies between countries. In the UK, if she is judged to be Fraser competent,[4] contraception, sexual health advice and treatment may be provided without parental knowledge or consent, although efforts should always be made to encourage her to discuss things with one or both parents, or another adult. It is important to ask sensitively about her relationship and to ensure that there is no coercion from her older partner. If any concerns are raised, the case could, in the first instance, be discussed with a colleague, bearing in mind that there is still a duty of confidentiality to the young person. If a health professional believes that there is a risk to the health, safety or welfare of the patient, which outweighs the right to privacy, locally agreed child protection procedures should be followed. It is essential, however, to try to establish a trusting relationship and encourage voluntary disclosure first.

How would you advise about sexually transmitted infections (STIs)?

Considerable rises in the incidence of STIs, particularly chlamydia, have led to a major public health problem in the UK.[1] Although rates in the under-16s have remained low, those in 16–19-year-olds and 20–24-year-olds almost trebled in men and more than doubled in women during the period 1995 to 2001. Gonorrhoea, and to a lesser extent genital herpes, have shown similar increases in incidence. It is therefore essential to discuss STIs and the use of condoms to help prevent infections. Early detection and treatment of curable STIs, such as chlamydia, can reduce the risk of further complications, such as infertility and ectopic pregnancy. She should also be advised to seek help should she develop symptoms such as a vaginal discharge.

What contraceptive methods would you advise?

The second National Survey of Sexual Attitudes and Lifestyles surveyed a total of 11 161 men and women aged 16–44 years between 1999 and 2001.[5] The proportion of those aged 16–19 years reporting first heterosexual intercourse at younger than 16 years was 30% for men and 26% for women, with a median age of 16 years. Non-use of contraception increased with declining age at first intercourse; 18% of men and 22% of women who had first intercourse at 13 or 14 years of age reported using no contraception. Early age of first intercourse was also significantly associated with pregnancy under age 18 years and a higher level of regret.

Every effort should be made to provide effective contraception and to encourage follow-up. They should be reassured that, if they have not yet had sex, starting a form of contraception should not make them feel pressurized to have intercourse before they feel ready.

All methods of contraception may be considered. Teenagers are relatively poor users of both barrier and hormonal contraceptives. Condoms remain the contraceptive of choice of young people; over 75% reported that they used condoms at their last sexual intercourse (15% reported using the oral contraceptive, 1% injectable contraception and 6% emergency contraception).[1] However, the combined use of condoms plus the contraceptive pill is probably the most effective option, as it protects against both pregnancy and STIs.

Emergency contraception is not a substitute for a regular form of contraception and does not protect against STIs. Access to emergency contraception, however, is an important and effective preventive measure against an unwanted pregnancy. However, as this patient is 14 years old, she may not be able to obtain it over the counter in pharmacies but may have to consult a health professional.

Recent Developments

1   While injectable contraceptives such as Depo-Provera are effective at reducing pregnancy, there are concerns about bone health.[6,7] The best available evidence suggests that the amenorrhoea induced by depot medroxyprogesterone acetate (DMPA) contraception is associated with a 5%–10% loss of bone, although it is not progressive. The long-term skeletal effects of DMPA in teenagers who have yet to achieve peak bone mass is presently uncertain and has to be balanced against the benefits of a very effective form of contraception. Any fall in bone mineral density (BMD) on starting treatment, however, seems to reverse rapidly on stopping DMPA.[8]

2   There is growing recognition that teenage pregnancy and early parenthood can lead to poor educational achievement, poor physical and mental health, poverty, and social isolation. European evidence has shown that a focus on the following may be effective in reducing the rate and negative consequences of teenage parenthood:[9]

    ●   improving contraceptive use and at least one other behaviour likely to prevent pregnancy and STI infection;

- providing long-term services and interventions tailored to meet local needs of young people, particularly in high-risk groups;

- providing clear and unambiguous information.

Conclusion

 It is important that this girl is given clear advice on the contraceptive methods suitable for her. She should be reassured that her parents do not need to know about the consultation. She should also be advised about the risks of developing sexually transmitted diseases.

Further Reading

1 Tripp J, Viner R. Sexual health, contraception, and teenage pregnancy. *BMJ* 2005; **330**: 590–3.

2 Santelli JS, Lindberg LD, Finer LB, Singh S. Explaining recent declines in adolescent pregnancy in the United States: the contribution of abstinence and improved contraceptive use. *Am J Public Health* 2007; **97**: 150–6.

3 Wilkinson P, French R, Kane R, Lachowycz K, Stephenson J, Grundy C, Jacklin P, Kingori P, Stevens M, Wellings K. Teenage conceptions, abortions, and births in England, 1994–2003, and the national teenage pregnancy strategy. *Lancet* 2006; **368**: 1879–86.

4 Samuels A. Contraception, pregnancy, childbirth – when things go wrong. *Med Sci Law* 1986; **26**: 39–47.

5 Wellings K, Nanchahal K, Macdowall W, McManus S, Erens B, Mercer CH, Johnson AM, Copas AJ, Korovessis C, Fenton KA, Field J. Sexual behaviour in Britain: early heterosexual experience. *Lancet* 2001; **358**: 1843–50.

6 World Health Organization (WHO). WHO Statement on Hormonal Contraception and Bone Health. July 2005. www.who.int/reproductive-health/family_planning/docs/hormonal_contraception_bone_health.pdf (accessed 19 09 07)

7 Rickert VI, Tiezzi L, Lipshutz J, León J, Vaughan RD, Westhoff C. Depo Now: preventing unintended pregnancies among adolescents and young adults. *J Adolesc Health* 2007; **40**: 22–8.

8 Scholes D, LaCroix AZ, Ichikawa LE, Barlow WE, Ott SM. Change in bone mineral density among adolescent women using and discontinuing depot medroxyprogesterone acetate contraception. *Arch Pediatr Adolesc Med* 2005; **159**: 139–44.

9 World Health Organization Regional office for Europe. Health Evidence Network (HEN). What are the most effective strategies for reducing the rate of teenage pregnancies? www.euro.who.int/HEN/Syntheses/short/20040423_6 (accessed 19 09 07)

25 Contraception after Age 35 Years

Case History

A 40-year-old lady requests contraceptive advice. She has recently started a relationship with a new partner of the same age. She has two children from a previous relationship and she is very sure that she does not wish to have any more children. During her previous relationship she took the combined oral contraceptive (COC) pill and this suited her well.

What are the important points to record in the history?

What are the choices available and which methods are most appropriate?

How long does she need to continue with contraception?

Background

Contraceptive choices for women over the age of 35 years differ from those of teenagers and younger women for a number of reasons. With increasing age, concurrent medical conditions are more likely to exist and risk–benefit ratios of the different methods often change. Frequency of intercourse, sexual function, menstrual irregularities and hormonal changes all impact on contraceptive choice.

Although there is a natural decline in fertility with age, pregnancy in older women is associated with a higher risk of miscarriage, congenital and chromosomal abnormalities, pregnancy complications and maternal morbidity and mortality.[1] Unwanted pregnancy leading to termination is often particularly distressing in this group of patients. It is therefore essential to offer an acceptable method which also provides effective contraceptive cover.

What are the important points to record in the history?

It is essential to take a careful medical history, with particular emphasis on cardiovascular risk factors, malignant disease and medication. Family history remains of importance, as does smoking status, and a brief obstetric and gynaecological history should be recorded, including date of the last cervical smear.

Often overlooked in this age group, but of particular importance, is the need to record a sexual history. The importance of using barrier contraception is often not appreciated in relationships in later life. Sterilization is more common, and having more often been in long-term relationships previously, the risk of sexually transmitted infection (STI) is often not considered seriously enough. As a result, the prevalence of STIs in this age group is increasing.[2]

What are the choices available and which methods are most appropriate?

The World Health Organization *Medical Eligibility Criteria for Contraceptive Use* (WHOMEC)[3] offers guidance on the safety of use of 19 different methods of contraception for women or men with specific characteristics or known medical conditions. The recommendations are based on systematic reviews of available clinical and epidemiological research. Categories include circumstances where generally the benefits of using a particular method outweigh the risks (WHO category 1: unrestricted use; and WHO category 2: benefits outweigh risks) and circumstances where the reverse is true (WHO category 3: risks outweigh the benefits, use with caution; and WHO category 4: use of the method poses an unacceptable health risk).

Combined hormonal contraception

The use of the combined oral contraceptive pill reduces with age, with 55% of 18- and 19-year-olds using it as their main method compared with just under one-third of women aged 30–34 years.[4] Eligibility depends largely on the presence of pre-existing disease or risk factors. The incidence of cardiovascular and cerebrovascular disease, although rare in women of reproductive age, rises with increasing age. Women who do not smoke and have no risk factors for cardiovascular or cerebrovascular disease may use the COC pill in WHO category 2. Women with pre-existing disease fall into WHO category 3 or 4.

The presence of risk factors such as hypertension or a significant family history of cardiovascular disease should raise concern and alternative methods of contraception should be considered. Smoking is an independent risk factor for cardiovascular and cerebrovascular disease and risk is further increased by the use of the COC pill. Furthermore, there is evidence that smoking increases the risk of venous thromboembolism, also higher in women taking the COC pill. For these reasons, use of the COC pill in women aged over 35 years who smoke more than 15 cigarettes a day is considered to be WHO category 4.

Migraine increases the risk of ischaemic stroke three-fold. COC pill users with migraine have a further increased risk. For this reason, WHOMEC recommends category 3 or 4 for women aged over 35 years with migraine, with or without aura.

The risk of breast cancer increases with increasing age. A meta-analysis of case–control studies showed a 24% increased background risk of breast cancer in women using the COC pill, which gradually returns to normal within ten years of stopping.[5] Clearly, background risk increases with age so it is important to counsel women regarding this risk.

Progesterone-only contraception

Risk factors associated with oestrogen mean that progesterone-only contraception (POC) is often more popular in women of increasing age. A WHO case–control study showed no increased risk of cardiovascular or cerebrovascular disease in normotensive women using oral or injectable progestogen but a ten-fold increased risk of stroke in hypertensive POC users.[6] Once again, WHOMEC[2] advises on the suitability of POC for women with existing medical conditions. Those with a personal history of ischaemic heart disease or stroke are advised that the risks of injectable POC outweigh the benefits and use is not recommended, although this does not apply to oral POC, implants or the levonorgestrel-releasing intrauterine system (LNG-IUS).

Other methods

Male or female sterilization is more popular in women over the age of 30 years who have completed their families. Use of copper-containing intrauterine devices is also popular, and if fitted after the age of 40 years, they may remain until contraception is no longer required.

Barrier methods or natural family planning are often chosen, although the higher failure rate of these methods should be emphasized. Use of condoms in all new relationships should be encouraged to minimize the risk of STIs.

How long does she need to continue with contraception?

The menopause is usually defined clinically after one year of amenorrhoea. Expert opinion advises that contraception should be continued until two years of amenorrhoea if aged under 50 years and one year if aged over 50 years. In general, most women will be menopausal and may discontinue contraception at the age of 55 years. Obviously, use of hormonal contraception, including the levonorgestrel-releasing intrauterine device, may make the assessment of amenorrhoea more difficult. Follicle-stimulating hormone (FSH) measurements are not a reliable indicator of ovarian failure, even if measured in the hormone-free interval.[1]

Recent Developments

1 There is much debate surrounding the use of injectable POC, principally the use of depot medroxyprogesterone acetate (DMPA) and bone health. The use of DMPA produces a hypo-oestrogenic state, and some studies have shown that this is associated with a decrease in bone mineral density (BMD).[7] Reduction in BMD seems to plateau after the first few years of use of DMPA and returns to that of comparable non-DMPA users over a period of 2–3 years. The effects appear to be reversible.[8] However, if women are using DMPA until their peri-menopausal years, there may not be sufficient time for bone density to return to normal before menopausal bone loss begins. This risk appears to be confined to injectable POC and is not relevant to other POC methods.

2 Use of the levonorgestrel-releasing intrauterine device is becoming increasingly popular and may be useful for older women with menorrhagia or those requiring hormone replacement therapy (see Cases 1: Menorrhagia with Medical Management and 11: Peri-menopausal Menstrual Symptoms).

Conclusion

Pregnancy in older women is likely to be complicated as they are more likely to have coexisting chronic medical conditions, particularly diabetes and hypertension. The risks of pregnancy complications, including pre-eclampsia and gestational diabetes, are significantly higher among older than among younger women, and ante-partum haemorrhage and placenta praevia are also more likely. A few women will die. The baby is more likely to be delivered by Caesarean section (either electively or because of an increased incidence of fetal distress) or by instrumental delivery, which, among parous older women, is more likely to be associated with post-partum haemorrhage. The risk of fetal malformation is also significantly related to age. Thus it is essential that this woman uses an effective form of contraception.[9]

Further Reading

1 Faculty of Family Planning and Reproductive Health Care Clinical Effectiveness Unit. FFPRHC Guidance (January 2005) Contraception for women aged over 40 years. *J Fam Plann Reprod Health Care* 2005; **31**: 51–64.

2 Centers for Disease Control and Prevention. Trends in Reportable Sexually Transmitted Diseases in the United States, 2005. www.cdc.gov (accessed 19 09 07)

3 World Health Organization (WHO). *Medical Eligibility Criteria for Contraceptive Use*, 3rd edn. Geneva: WHO Press, 2004.

4 Dawe F, Rainford L. *Contraception and Sexual Health, 2003.* London: Office for National Statistics, 2003; 1–54.

5 Collaborative Group on Hormonal Factors in Breast Cancer. Breast cancer and hormonal contraceptives: collaborative reanalysis of individual data on 53 297 women with breast cancer and 100 239 women without breast cancer from 54 epidemiological studies. *Lancet* 1996; **347**: 1713–27.

6 World Health Organization Collaborative Study of Cardiovascular Disease and Steroid Hormone Contraception. Cardiovascular disease and use of oral and injectable progestogen-only contraceptives and combined injectable contraceptives. Results of an international, multicenter, case–control study. *Contraception* 1998; **57**: 315–24.

7 World Health Organization. WHO Statement on Hormonal Contraception and Bone Health. July 2005. www.who.int/reproductive-health/family_planning/docs/hormonal_contraception_bone_health.pdf (accessed 19 09 07)

8 Scholes D, LaCroix AZ, Ichikawa LE, Barlow WE, Ott SM. Injectable hormone contraception and bone density: results from a prospective study. *Epidemiology* 2002; **13**: 581–7.

9 Glasier A. Pregnancy in women over 45: should this be encouraged? *Menopause Int* 2007; **13**: 6–7.

Gynaecological Emergencies

26 Early Miscarriage

Case History

A 39-year-old woman with three children has been using the progesterone-only pill for contraception for two years. She has not missed any pills but feels unmistakably pregnant. With this form of contraception, her periods are usually irregular but she has had no bleeding for eight weeks. She now has bleeding like a period and also mild constant pain in her right iliac fossa. A pregnancy test is positive. An ultrasound scan reveals an empty uterus with a thin endometrium and normal adnexae with no free fluid. Serum human chorionic gonadotrophin (hCG) level is 215 IU/l. Repeat serum hCG 48 hours later is 49 IU/l.

How can one distinguish an ectopic pregnancy from an early intrauterine pregnancy or from a complete miscarriage?

What treatment options are open to her once a diagnosis is made?

What advice should be given to women following a miscarriage?

Background

Miscarriage is defined as the loss of an intrauterine pregnancy before viability (24 weeks), but most miscarriages occur in the first trimester. Clinicians should avoid using negative terminology such as 'pregnancy failure'. 'Abortion', an old medical term used to mean pregnancy loss, should not be used in this context. Miscarriage in the first trimester is very common, with approximately one in six clinical pregnancies ending in miscarriage.[1]

How can one distinguish an ectopic pregnancy from an early intrauterine pregnancy or from a miscarriage?

Using transvaginal ultrasound scanning (TVS), it is usually possible to detect an intrauterine pregnancy sac with a yolk sac from five weeks following the last normal menstrual period (Figure 26.1). If the gestational sac is greater than 20 mm in diameter, a fetal pole or a yolk sac should be visible. At six weeks, the fetal pole should be visible and a fetal heart can usually be detected. If the fetal pole is greater than 6 mm in length, a fetal heart should be visible. The absence of these signs at six weeks does not necessarily mean that the pregnancy is non-viable and a repeat scan is usually arranged for one week later. This has been termed a pregnancy of uncertain viability.

Until a pregnancy is definitely seen within the uterus, doubt remains as to its location. This has been termed a pregnancy of unknown location. At this point, a single serum hCG measurement can be taken to estimate the likely size of the pregnancy. A pregnancy with serum hCG above approximately 1500–2000 IU/l should be visible within the

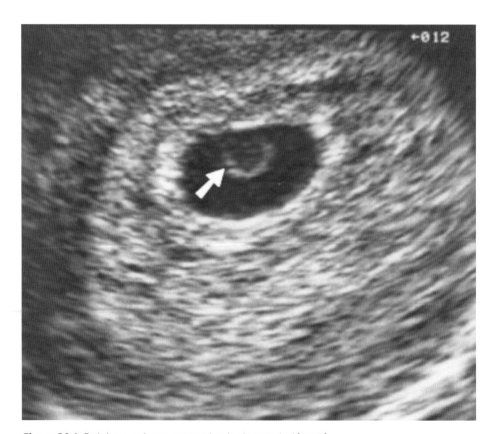

Figure 26.1 Early intrauterine pregnancy showing 'cygnet ring' (arrow).

uterus. In a healthy pregnancy, the serum level of hCG should increase by at least two-thirds every 48 hours from about five to eight weeks. Clearly, in a failing pregnancy of whatever location, hCG levels will remain static or fall. Ectopic pregnancies may still rupture with hCG levels below 1000 IU/l.

In some units, serum progesterone measurement is used to try to identify pregnancies destined to fail. A level above 60 nmol/l is associated with a viable pregnancy. A pregnancy with levels below 20 nmol/l is likely to miscarry safely, whatever its location.[2]

What treatment options are open to her once a diagnosis is made?

Having choice over the management of miscarriage is associated with better health-related quality of life.[3]

Expectant management allows nature to take its course. If bleeding is already quite heavy, this is probably the best option and is associated with more than 90% complete resolution of symptoms for incomplete miscarriage. If the patient has not yet started to bleed (a 'silent' miscarriage) she may still choose a conservative approach, but in a meta-analysis of 13 trials, only 28% of women completed their miscarriage without further intervention.[4]

Some women prefer a surgical approach and opt for an evacuation of retained products of conception (ERPC), which is usually done under general anaesthetic as a day case. If the woman is bleeding extremely heavily and persistently, an emergency ERPC may be required. Other positive indications for ERPC include associated infection and suspected molar pregnancy. ERPC carries a complication rate of approximately 2%.[5] The most common complications are retained products of conception and infection (both of which may also occur with expectant and medical management). Uterine perforation can occur following ERPC, but damage to the cervix by forced dilation is rare and can be reduced by preparing the cervix with misoprostol.

In women whose blood group is Rhesus negative, anti-D immunoglobulin should be given in the following circumstances: all miscarriages over twelve weeks, ectopic pregnancy, following ERPC and if bleeding is heavy or painful. Guidelines suggest that all women who are going to have an ERPC should be screened for chlamydia infection in order to reduce the incidence of ascending pelvic infection.[1]

What advice should be given to women following a miscarriage?

Bleeding following a miscarriage may last up to three weeks. If she continues to get pain or bleeding or to have an offensive discharge she should seek medical advice.

Women very commonly wish to establish why the miscarriage has occurred and often blame themselves for it. The vast majority of miscarriages occur because there was a fundamental abnormality with the developing pregnancy: chromosomal abnormality can be detected in over 50% of products of conception.[6] It may be reassuring for her to know that it is not her fault and that there was nothing she could have done to prevent it.

Recent Developments

Medical management of miscarriage should be available. A number of regimens are used but usually involve an oral or vaginal prostaglandin analogue and possibly the anti-progesterone, mifepristone. Treatment can be taken at home, but women must be given high-quality advice and have access to 24-hour hospital admission. In the management of incomplete miscarriage, medical and surgical treatments appear equally effective but medical management is associated with a significantly lower rate of infection.[7]

Conclusion

If the couple wish to try to become pregnant again, they are usually advised to wait for two or three normal cycles first. This is partly to allow the body to recover physically and to demonstrate that the miscarriage is complete before embarking on a further pregnancy. However, the two or three months can also be important to allow them to recover emotionally before starting again. If they happen to conceive sooner than that, there should be no adverse consequences for the pregnancy.

Further Reading

1 Royal College of Obstetricians and Gynaecologists (RCOG). *The Management of Early Pregnancy Loss*. Green-top Guideline No. 25. London: RCOG Press, 2006.

2 Banerjee S, Aslam N, Woelfer B, Lawrence A, Elson J, Jurkovic D. Expectant management of early pregnancies of unknown location: a prospective evaluation of methods to predict spontaneous resolution of pregnancy. *BJOG* 2001; 108: 158–63.

3 Wieringa-De Waard M, Hartman E, Ankum W, Reitsma J, Bindels P, Bonsel G. Expectant management versus surgical evacuation in first trimester miscarriage: health-related quality of life in randomized and non-randomized patients. *Hum Reprod* 2002; 17: 1638–42.

4 Graziosi GC, Mol BW, Ankum WM, Bruinse HW. Management of early pregnancy loss. *Int J Gynecol Obstet* 2004; 86: 337–46.

5 Lawson HW, Frye A, Atrash HK, Smith JC, Shulman HB, Ramick M. Abortion mortality, United States, 1972 through 1987. *Am J Obstet Gynecol* 1994; 171: 1365–72.

6 Menasha J, Levy B, Hirschhorn K, Kardon NB. Incidence and spectrum of chromosome abnormalities in spontaneous abortions: new insights from a 12-year study. *Genet Med* 2005; 7: 251–63.

7 Demetroulis C, Saridogan E, Kunde D, Naftalin AA. A prospective randomized control trial comparing medical and surgical treatment for early pregnancy failure. *Hum Reprod* 2001; 16: 365–9.

27 Ectopic Pregnancy

Case History

A 32-year-old woman, who has been trying to conceive for 13 months, presents with seven weeks of amenorrhoea and bleeding like a light period. She has mild pain in the right iliac fossa. Transvaginal ultrasound scanning (TVS) shows a thickened endometrium, no intrauterine gestational sac, but free fluid in the pelvis. Serum human chorionic gonadotrophin (hCG) level is 2749 IU/l. Emergency laparoscopy and a salpingectomy are performed to remove a rupturing ectopic pregnancy.

What factors predispose an individual to ectopic pregnancy?

How does a typical ectopic pregnancy present and evolve?

Under what circumstance would one attempt to preserve the affected tube and how likely is she to achieve a successful pregnancy in future?

Background

An ectopic pregnancy is one implanted outside the uterine cavity, and 95% of such pregnancies are tubal. However, ectopic pregnancies can implant in the ovary, the omentum, the abdominal wall or the cervix. Typically, tubal pregnancies present at six to seven weeks, but pregnancies in more unusual locations tend to present later in the pregnancy and, particularly for the abdominal sites, may not present until term. Rarely, a multiple pregnancy may implant in two different sites. This is termed a heterotopic pregnancy and occurs spontaneously approximately once in 10 000 pregnancies. Following *in vitro* fertilization (IVF) the incidence is much higher, perhaps as high as 1 in 500 pregnancies.[1]

What factors predispose an individual to ectopic pregnancy?

Any event which leads to tubal damage or altered tubal transport will increase the risk of tubal pregnancy (Table 27.1). A history of ectopic pregnancy increases the risk of a second ectopic, with a 10% risk of ectopic in subsequent pregnancy. Tubal damage may occur as a result of pelvic infection, particularly chlamydia, or as a result of abdominal surgery, particularly tubal surgery. A history of subfertility may pre-date the ectopic, and IVF is associated with an increased risk of tubal pregnancy. Conception while taking the progesterone-only pill increases the risk. The copper intrauterine contraceptive device does not increase the absolute risk of ectopic pregnancy but it will not prevent implantation within the tube. Thus, if a pregnancy occurs with a copper device *in situ*, it is more

Table 27.1 Risk factors for tubal pregnancy
Previous tubal pregnancy
Previous tubal surgery, including reversal of sterilization
Previous pelvic infection, especially chlamydia
History of subfertility
In vitro fertilization
Progesterone-only contraceptive pill
Intrauterine contraceptive device

likely to be an ectopic pregnancy. Levonorgestrel-releasing devices are associated with a very low failure rate, but of these resulting pregnancies approximately half will be ectopic.[2]

How does a typical ectopic pregnancy present and evolve?

The diagnosis of ectopic pregnancy can be extremely difficult and it may present with a huge range of symptoms or none at all.

The presentation may be very dramatic, with collapse, but more commonly there is persistent pain of increasing intensity on one side or the other. There may be shoulder tip pain or syncope. Vaginal bleeding may be light or absent and may be fresh or dark. Heavy vaginal bleeding is more in keeping with miscarriage of an intrauterine pregnancy. Vaginal examination should always be performed at some point during the assessment to estimate uterine size and adnexal tenderness but it may be best for this to be done once and in a hospital setting.

The tools used to make the diagnosis are described in Case 26: Early Miscarriage. While ultrasound technology is improving, and the likelihood of positively identifying an ectopic pregnancy on scan increases, the definitive test is still a diagnostic laparoscopy (Figure 27.1). Treatment can be performed at the same operation. Laparoscopy itself is not without risk, carrying about a 1 in 500 risk of complications such as bowel damage, bleeding or infection. Laparoscopy is the operation of choice rather than laparotomy because recovery time and hospital stay are significantly reduced, with most patients going home the following day. However in a shocked patient, laparotomy may be appropriate in order to control bleeding as rapidly as possible.

Under what circumstance would one attempt to preserve the affected tube and how likely is she to achieve a successful pregnancy in future?

If the contralateral tube is normal, guidelines recommend that the tube containing the ectopic pregnancy is removed: salpingectomy.[3] Although intrauterine pregnancy rates may be slightly lower following salpingectomy rather than salpingotomy (hazard ratio 0.63; 95% confidence interval [CI] 0.421–0.940), removing the tube reduces the risk of subsequent ectopic pregnancy and of persistent trophoblastic tissue.[4] The cumulative spontaneous pregnancy rate at one year is 56% in women following salpingectomy and 72% following salpingotomy.[5]

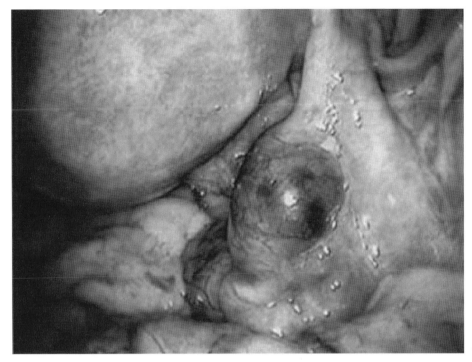

Figure 27.1 Laparoscopic image of an ectopic pregnancy.

If the contralateral tube is already damaged or absent, it may be possible to preserve the tube containing the ectopic pregnancy by removing the pregnancy through a linear incision: linear salpingotomy. In this case, the patient must be followed-up with serial serum hCG measurements to ensure that all the placental tissue has been removed. After treatment, the tube may heal and recanalize sufficiently to achieve a pregnancy.

Recent Developments

An ectopic pregnancy may miscarry spontaneously and need no specific treatment. However, if trophoblastic tissue appears to be continuing to proliferate (i.e. the serum hCG levels are rising or failing to fall adequately), it may be appropriate to treat the pregnancy with methotrexate. Medical treatment is probably inappropriate in women with serum hCG levels over 3000 IU/l, where fetal cardiac activity is seen or where a large adnexal mass or haemoperitoneum is present, because of the need to control or prevent bleeding. Methotrexate kills rapidly dividing cells and, given in a single or repeated intramuscular dose related to body surface area, is well tolerated. Pain may increase after the methotrexate has been administered and some women will still require surgery, but this intervention rate is less than 10% with appropriate patient selection. Medical treatment should only be used where staff are familiar with its use and it must be monitored using serial hCG measurements followed to a level below 20 IU/l. The patient should not conceive for three months following treatment (Royal College of Obstetricians and

Gynaecologists) but intrauterine pregnancy rates of over 50% at the end of the first year have been reported.[3,6]

Conclusion

Ectopic pregnancy accounts for 5% of maternal deaths in the developed world.[7,8] When speaking with the patient after the event, it is important to remember that she has both faced a life-threatening illness but also lost a pregnancy. The balance between these two sources of grief will vary according to her experience and her hopes for the future.

Further Reading

1 Serour GI, Aboulghar M, Mansour R, Sattar MA, Amin Y, Aboulghar H. Complications of medically assisted conception in 3,500 cycles. *Fertil Steril* 1998; **70**: 638–42.

2 Backman T, Rauramo I, Huhtala S, Koskenvuo M. Pregnancy during the use of levonorgestrel intrauterine system. *Am J Obstet Gynecol* 2004; **190**: 50–4.

3 Royal College of Obstetricians and Gynaecologists (RCOG). *The Management of Tubal Pregnancy*. Green-top Guideline No. 21. London: RCOG Press, 2004.

4 Bangsgaard N, Lund C, Ottesen B, Nilas L. Improved fertility following conservative surgical treatment of ectopic pregnancy. *BJOG* 2003; **110**: 765–70.

5 Job-Spira N, Bouyer J, Pouly J, Germain E, Coste J, Aublet-Cuvelier B, Fernandez H. Fertility after ectopic pregnancy: first results of a population-based cohort study in France. *Hum Reprod* 1996; **11**: 99–104.

6 Gervaise A, Masson L, de Tayrac R, Frydman R, Fernandez H. Reproductive outcome after methotrexate treatment of tubal pregnancies. *Fertil Steril* 2004; **82**: 304–8.

7 Sowter MC, Farquhar CM. Ectopic pregnancy: an update. *Curr Opin Obstet Gynecol* 2004; **16**: 289–93.

8 Khan KS, Wojdyla D, Say L, Gülmezoglu AM, Van Look PF. WHO analysis of causes of maternal death: a systematic review. *Lancet* 2006; **367**: 1066–74.

28 Hydatidiform Mole

Case History

A 26-year-old woman,15 weeks pregnant, is admitted to hospital with vaginal bleeding. She is very anxious and complains of palpitations. Her vital signs are blood pressure 190/110 mmHg, pulse rate 112 beats per minute and respiration rate 22 per minute. On physical examination, her uterus is large for dates. The laboratory findings are haemoglobin 9 g/100 ml, white cell count 8000×10^6 cells/l, platelets $160\ 000 \times 10^6$ cells/l, free T3 (triiodothyronine) highly elevated, free T4 (thyroxine) highly elevated, thyroid-stimulating hormone (TSH) <0.01 mU/l, and serum human chorionic gonadotrophin (hCG) 250 000 mIU/ml.

How do you investigate?

How do you manage this patient?

What is the proper follow-up after hydatidiform mole evacuation?

What is the impact of a hydatidiform mole on subsequent pregnancies?

What if the serum hCG level does not normalize after molar evacuation?

Background

How do you investigate?

Abnormally elevated serum hCG levels, vaginal bleeding and an excessively enlarged uterus point to the diagnosis of hydatidiform mole. However, an hCG value in the normal range does not exclude it. The work-up should include a complete blood count and coagulation profile, renal- and liver-function tests and thyroid function tests. An ultrasound scan is performed to confirm diagnosis and in most cases identifies a hydatidiform mole as a complex intrauterine mass with multiple anechoic areas of varying size (snowstorm appearance; Figure 28.1). An ultrasound scan may also find a twin pregnancy where there is one viable fetus and the other pregnancy is molar. In the latter case, the pregnancy can be allowed to proceed if the mother wishes, following appropriate counselling.[1] A chest X-ray should be taken once the diagnosis of a hydatidiform mole has been made.

How do you manage this patient?

Patients with molar pregnancies may suffer from various medical complications including hyperthyroidism, hyperemesis gravidarum, pre-eclampsia, trophoblastic embolization

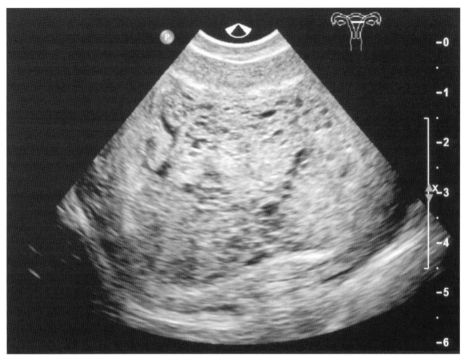

Figure 28.1 Transabdominal ultrasonography of a molar pregnancy: the uterus is bulky and the endometrial cavity is filled with an echogenic structure containing multiple small cysts.

and theca lutein ovarian cysts (Table 28.1). Consequently, symptoms can vary and include hypertension, proteinuria, hyper-reflexia indicating pre-eclampsia, palpitations, weight loss and tremor caused by hyperthyroidism, abdominal pain from theca lutein ovarian cysts which can tort or rupture (leading to an acute abdomen), and respiratory

Table 28.1 Symptoms and complications of a hydatidiform mole
Vaginal bleeding
Excessive uterine size
Theca lutein ovarian cysts   Ovarian torsion, cyst rupture, acute abdomen
Pre-eclampsia   Hypertension, proteinuria, hyper-reflexia
Hyperemesis
Hyperthyroidism   Palpitations, tremor, weight loss
Trophoblastic emboli   Respiratory distress

distress due to trophoblastic embolization. Some complications are potentially life-threatening and consideration should be given to treat a mole in a facility with an intensive care unit.

Hydatidiform moles should be evacuated as soon as possible after stabilization of any medical complications. Heavy vaginal bleeding secondary to a molar pregnancy may require immediate attention, including resuscitation with blood transfusions.

Suction curettage followed by blunt curettage of the uterine cavity is the method of choice for the evacuation of a hydatidiform mole. Ripening of the cervix with prostanoids prior to suction evacuation should be avoided as it might promote dissemination of trophoblastic cells. Similarly, there is a theoretical concern over the routine use of oxytocic agents during evacuation because of the potential to embolize trophoblastic tissue through the venous system. Therefore it is recommended, where possible, that oxytocin infusions are commenced once evacuation has been completed.[1] If oxytocin is ineffective to control peri-operative hemorrhage, prostaglandin analogues or oxytocics such as ergometrine may be administered. Rhesus-negative patients should be treated with anti-D immunoglobulin after evacuation.[2]

All tissue obtained during evacuation should undergo histological examination. After final diagnosis is made, patients should be registered with a trophoblastic disease centre.

It is important to control thyroid function prior to the induction of anaesthesia for molar evacuation because the surgery may precipitate a thyroid storm, characterized by hyperthermia, convulsions, atrial fibrillation or high-output cardiac failure. Symptoms of hyperthyroidism are successfully treated by β-blockers such as propranolol. The use of thyrostatic agents like methimazole or propylthiouracil may also be required.

In patients who do not wish further childbearing, a total abdominal hysterectomy with the molar pregnancy *in situ* can be considered. Hysterectomy reduces the risk of malignant post-molar sequelae compared with evacuation by vacuum curettage. However, the risk of persistent gestational trophoblastic disease after hysterectomy remains.

What is the proper follow-up after hydatidiform mole evacuation?

Follow-up with regular measurement of serum hCG levels is essential after evacuation of a molar pregnancy. It is used to detect persistent disease and to determine who will require further treatment. A baseline serum hCG level should be checked within 48 hours of evacuation. Tests of serum hCG levels are then performed weekly until undetectable levels have been obtained for three consecutive weeks, and then monthly for twelve months.

During the surveillance period contraception is required because pregnancy would obviate the usefulness of serum hCG as a tumour marker. Oral contraceptive pills are a safe and effective choice.[3]

What is the impact of a hydatidiform mole on subsequent pregnancies?

In general, once a 6–12-month surveillance establishes a disease-free status, conception can be considered, although women with a history of trophoblastic disease have a 10-fold increased risk (1–2% incidence) for future molar disease and will require close observation during future pregnancies.[2,4] A pelvic ultrasound examination should be performed during the first trimester of all subsequent pregnancies to confirm that gestation is normal. Furthermore, the serum hCG level should be checked six weeks after completion of the pregnancy to exclude occult trophoblastic disease.

What if the serum hCG level does not normalize after molar evacuation?

Patients with (a) four values or more of plateau ± 10% serum hCG levels over three weeks, (b) a rise of serum hCG level of 10% or greater for three values over two weeks, or (c) elevated serum hCG values six months after evacuation, are most likely suffering from persistent trophoblastic neoplasia, and should be referred to an experienced centre for appropriate treatment.[5]

Recent Developments

In the months following evacuation of a hydatidiform mole some patients might develop persistent low hCG results. Although false-positive serum hCG levels are rare, they have led clinicians to perform unnecessary medical interventions, including chemotherapies and hysterectomies. False-positive hCG occurs when human heterophilic antibodies in the circulation interfere with hCG tests, cross-linking antibodies. It is characterized by:

● widely varying hCG results in different hCG tests;

● negative urine hCG;

● non-parallel quantitative serum results when the sample is diluted, and

● successful blocking of serum reactivity using heterophilic antibody blocking agents.

Another reason for persistant low hCG results is quiescent gestational trophoblastic disease (GTD), a benign form of trophoblastic disease marked by the absence of cytotrophoblast cells, the invasive or malignant cell component. Hyperglycosylated hCG (hCG-H) in serum of patients aids in the differential diagnosis of quiescent GTD and persistant trophoblastic neoplasia. It marks the presence of invasive trophoblast cells and is the predominant form of hCG in the circulation of patients with persistant trophoblastic neoplasia or choriocarcinomas. It is not prominent in benign cases of hydatidiform mole or quiescent GTD.[5]

Conclusion

The patient's thyrotoxicosis is treated with methimazole and propanolol to achieve haemodynamic stability before surgery. She then undergoes an uncomplicated suction curettage. The per vaginal bleeding stops and the baseline serum hCG level after 48 hours is 95 000 mIU/ml. She is put on a contraceptive pill and has weekly tests of serum hCG levels which become undetectable after 8 weeks. They remain undetectable for three consecutive weeks, after which the patient is followed up with monthly serum hCG levels for 10 months. At this stage the patient has a strong desire to fall pregnant and stops taking the contraceptive pill. She falls pregnant 2 months later. A pelvic ultrasound at 8 weeks confirms a viable intrauterine pregnancy and excludes a hydatidiform mole.

Management of a hydatidiform mole

Investigations

- Quantitative serum hCG
- Ultrasound examination
- Full blood count
- Coagulation studies
- Liver and renal function tests
- Thyroid function tests
- Blood group with antibody screen
- Chest X-ray

Treatment

- Management of medical complications
- Uterine evacuation with post-operative oxytocics
- Anti-D immunoglobulin for Rhesus-negative patients after evacuation

Follow-up

- Serum hCG surveillance for 6–12 months
- Contraception for 6–12 months

Further Reading

1 Royal College of Obstetricians and Gynaecologists (RCOG). *The Management of Gestational Trophoblastic Neoplasia.* Green-top Guideline No. 38. London: RCOG Press, 2004.

2 Soper JT, Mutch DG, Schink JC. Diagnosis and treatment of gestational trophoblastic disease: ACOG Practice Bulletin No. 53. *Gynecol Oncol* 2004; **93**: 575–85.

3 Gerulath AH, Ehlen TG, Bessette P, Jolicoeur L, Savoie R. Gestational trophoblastic disease. *J Obstet Gynaecol Can* 2002; **24**: 434–46.

4 Garner EI, Lipson E, Bernstein MR, Goldstein DP, Berkowitz RS. Subsequent pregnancy experience in patients with molar pregnancy and gestational trophoblastic tumor. *J Reprod Med* 2002; **47**: 380–6.

5 Khanlian SA, Cole LA. Management of gestational trophoblastic disease and other cases with low serum levels of human chorionic gonadotropin. *J Reprod Med* 2006; **51**: 812–18.

29 Emergency Contraception

History

A 17-year-old woman requests emergency contraception on a Monday morning. She has been sexually active with her new partner for the past few weeks and had unprotected sexual intercourse (UPSI) two days ago. Her last menstrual period was three weeks ago.

What are the two main methods of emergency contraception?

What is their mode of action?

Which factors would help you to decide which method to use?

What additional questions would you like to ask?

What are the important aspects of follow-up?

Background

What are the two main methods of emergency contraception?

The purpose of emergency contraception is to provide women with a safe means of preventing pregnancy following either unprotected sexual intercourse (UPSI) or potential contraceptive failure.[1]

The two main methods currently available are the progesterone pill, containing 1.5 mg levonorgestrel (LNG), which is given as a single dose, and the copper-containing intrauterine contraceptive device (IUCD). The most commonly used method is the LNG-containing pill and this is licensed to be given within 72 hours of unprotected intercourse, although it is known to have some efficacy for up to 120 hours after UPSI.[2] The sooner the pill is administered, the greater the efficacy. Despite the fact that the LNG-containing pill is now readily available in pharmacies in countries such as the United Kingdom (UK), its use amongst women requesting termination of pregnancy (TOP) remains low (1% in 1984, 6% in 1996 and 12% in 2002).[3] The IUCD is the more effective of the two methods. Insertion of a copper IUCD is effective up to 120 hours (five days) after intercourse, or up to five days after the earliest possible date of ovulation (ovulation occurs 14 days prior to menstruation). The LNG-containing intrauterine device is not recommended.

What is their mode of action?

The mode of action of oral LNG is incompletely understood but appears to relate to prevention of ovulation, rather than inhibition of implantation.[1] The mechanism of action of the IUCD is clearer and relates to the direct toxicity of the copper contained within the device. This produces pre- and post-fertilization effects.[4] It may be inserted up to five days after the most likely date of ovulation and, if given at this time, will produce an inflammatory reaction within the endometrium, preventing implantation.[5] If given earlier in the cycle, its principal action is to prevent fertilization, and alterations in the copper content of the cervical mucus probably also inhibit sperm penetration.[5]

Which factors would help you to decide which method to use?

The date of the last menstrual period and whether it was in any way abnormal are crucial in determining which method of emergency contraception to offer (Figure 29.1) Not only does this allow you to assess the risk of pregnancy but it also impacts on the ability to offer an IUCD according to the expected date of ovulation.

UPSI on or around day 14 of a 28-day cycle carries a higher risk of pregnancy, and an IUCD would be the method of choice because of its higher efficacy.

What additional questions would you like to ask?

It is important to ask whether this was a single act of UPSI or if there have been multiple episodes in this cycle. If there have been other episodes, more than 72 hours ago, and if she has already taken the LNG-containing pill earlier in her cycle, its use is now off licence.[6] This must be explained to her, as well as making it clear that there is no evidence

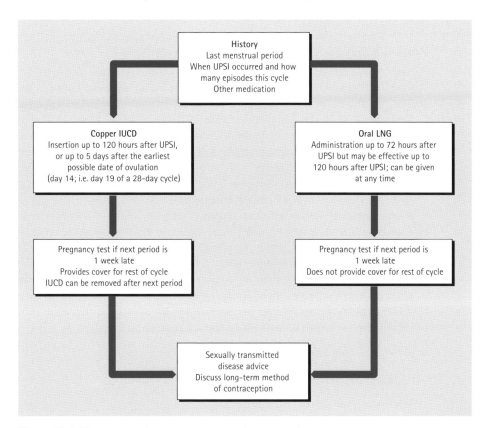

Figure 29.1 Management of emergency contraception.

that the method will have any effect on preventing pregnancy which may have occurred as a result of previous episodes of UPSI.

It is important to take a brief medical history, particularly to ascertain whether she is taking any other medication. Liver enzyme-inducing drugs (including the herbal remedy St John's wort) have the potential to reduce efficacy of the LNG method so an IUCD should be offered as an alternative, or the dose of LNG should be increased to a total of 3 mg, although, once again, this is outside the product licence.[1] There is also potential for LNG to antagonize the anticoagulant effect of phenindione and warfarin,[7] so special attention should be paid to monitoring anticoagulation following administration.

The World Health Organization *Medical Eligibility Criteria for Contraceptive Use*[8] states that there are no absolute medical contraindications to the use of LNG as emergency contraception, although the UK British National Formulary advises caution with a history of ectopic pregnancy, severe malabsorption syndromes, severe liver disease, or pregnancy and breast-feeding.[7] Clearly, a known sensitivity to progesterone should also raise concern.

Absolute contraindications to the use of a copper-containing IUCD are few and are the same as those for routine IUCD use.[9] The use of routine prophylactic antibiotics has been shown to confer little benefit,[10] although should be considered in women at high risk of sexually transmitted infections (STIs). Choice of antibiotic should be based on advice from local genitourinary services and should cover the possibility of asymptomatic chlamydia infection.

What are the important aspects of follow-up?

Having given a full explanation of both methods and administered emergency contraception, in this case the LNG-containing pill, there are a number of important follow-up points.

No method of emergency contraception is 100% effective, so the patient should be advised to return for a pregnancy test if her next period is a week late. She should also be advised that LNG emergency contraception does not provide cover for the rest of the cycle.

Future contraception should be considered and it may be appropriate to begin a long-term method, such as Depo-Provera or the combined oral contraceptive (COC) pill, either immediately or with the next normal period.

Women starting hormonal contraception without waiting for a period should be advised regarding the length of time before the method becomes protective against pregnancy and a follow-up pregnancy test should always be arranged. Women who choose the IUCD as their method of emergency contraception may have the device removed after their next normal period, or they may decide to keep it as ongoing contraception.

Finally, a sexual history should always be obtained and guidance regarding screening for STIs should be given. The use of condoms to reduce the risk of infection should also be encouraged.

Recent Developments

Mifepristone can also be used for emergency contraception.[11,12] It probably acts by inhibiting or delaying ovulation. A single dose of 600 mg mifepristone within 72 h of unprotected intercourse has been shown to be more effective than the traditional Yuzpe regimen in preventing pregnancy. The incidence of side effects with mifepristone was also significantly lower than that of the Yuzpe regimen. A subsequent multicentre randomized comparative study showed that a dose as low as 10 mg was already effective as an emergency contraceptive. No major side effects occurred but the delay in return of menstruation was significantly related to the dose of mifepristone which could increase anxiety. As 10 mg of mifepristone is not abortifacient, this may help to improve the acceptability of the drug as an emergency contraceptive. However, the use of mifepristone as an abortion drug may limit its availability in countries where abortion is not legal.

Conclusion

In this case, the patient has now reached day 21, and is thus more than five days after the earliest possible date for ovulation. Thus the LNG-containing pill should be offered. She is adamant she does not want the problem to happen again and has elected for Depo-Provera for future contraception and will also use condoms to prevent sexually transmitted diseases.

Further Reading

1 Faculty of Family Planning and Reproductive Health Care Clinical Effectiveness Unit. FFPRHC Guidance (April 2006). Emergency contraception. *J Fam Plann Reprod Health Care* 2006; **32**: 121–8.

2 von Hertzen H, Piaggio G, Ding J, Chen J, Song S, Bartfai G, Ng E, Gemzell-Danielsson K, Oyunbileg A, Wu S, Cheng W, Ludicke F, Pretnar-Darovec A, Kirkman R, Mittal S, Khomassuridze A, Apter D, Peregoudov A. Low-dose mifepristone and two regimens of levonorgestrel for emergency contraception: a WHO multicentre randomised trial. *Lancet* 2002; **360**: 1803–10.

3 Glasier A. Emergency contraception. Is it worth all the fuss? *BMJ* 2006; **333**: 560–1.

4 Stanford JB, Mikolajczyk RT. Mechanisms of action of intrauterine devices: update and estimation of postfertilization effects. *Am J Obstet Gynecol* 2002; **187**: 1699–708.

5 Ortiz ME, Croxatto HB, Bardin CW. Mechanisms of action of intrauterine devices. *Obstet Gynecol Surv* 1996; **51** (12 Suppl): S42–51.

6 Faculty of Family Planning and Reproductive Health Care Clinical Effectiveness Unit. FFPRHC Guidance (July 2005). The use of contraception outside the terms of the product licence. *J Fam Plann Reprod Health Care* 2005; **31**: 225–42.

7 British Medical Association and the Royal Pharmaceutical Society of Great Britain. *British National Formulary*, Vol. 53. March 2007.

8 World Health Organization (WHO). *Medical Eligibility Criteria for Contraceptive Use*, 3rd edn. Geneva: WHO Press, 2004.

9 Faculty of Family Planning and Reproductive Health Care Clinical Effectiveness Unit. FFPRHC Guidance (January 2004). The copper intrauterine device as long-term contraception. *J Fam Plann Reprod Health Care* 2004; **30**: 29–42.

10 Grimes DA, Schulz KF. Antibiotic prophylaxis for intrauterine contraceptive device insertion. *Cochrane Database Syst Rev* 2001; CD001327.

11 Tang OS, Ho PC. Clinical applications of mifepristone. *Gynecol Endocrinol* 2006; 22: 655–9.

12 Cheng L, Gulmezoglu AM, Oel CJ, Piaggio G, Ezcurra E, Look PF. Interventions for emergency contraception. *Cochrane Database Syst Rev* 2004; CD001324.

Sexual Problems

30 Lack of Sex Drive

Case History

A 53-year-old woman mentions in passing that her interest in sex has fallen since her periods stopped a year ago. She and her 55-year-old partner, with whom she has been in a stable relationship for 25 years, are unhappy about this.

What do you do?

How do you assess the situation?

What is your management plan?

Background

Sexual problems are frequent in menopausal women.[1] Ageing and length of the relationship with a partner are known to affect sexual function of both sexes. The longitudinal Melbourne Women's Midlife Health Project found a highly significant negative effect of ageing on frequency of sexual activity, sexual interest (libido), and aspects of sexual responsiveness, sexual arousal, enjoyment, and orgasm.[2] Furthermore, a number of studies have found an additional decrement in aspects of sexual function in midlife, coinciding with the menopause.

What do you do?

The problem has been mentioned at the end of the consultation and it would be advisable to find out if this is something she wants to discuss with you further. She may want to come alone initially and then with her partner. Before the next consultation it would be prudent to review the medical and social histories of both partners, if available, for any long-standing underlying problems.

How do you assess the situation?

The aim of the consultation is to try and identify the main problem, whether it be male or female:

- decreased or absent sexual desire (loss of libido) in either partner
- arousal disorders
- lack or loss of orgasm
- painful intercourse
- vaginismus
- erectile dysfunction
- premature or retarded ejaculation
- sexual violence
- others, such as fear of a sexually transmitted disease, gender confusion and paraphilias (abnormal sexual activity that is socially prohibited)

There are now international definitions and classifications of the various types of female sexual dysfunction (Table 30.1).[3]

It is important to find out the duration of the problem, how often intercourse occurs, is the relationship monogamous, the sexual orientation of both partners (straight, gay, bisexual) and if there are problems within the relationship(s). Since sexual problems may be part of an ongoing illness or a side effect of treatment (such as with antihypertensives or antidepressants), or occur as a result of disability, this needs to be ascertained in both partners. Confidentiality has to be maintained; it cannot be assumed that the couple have informed each other of any medical problems.

Further assessment depends on the result of the initial interview. She should be offered an examination. If there are concerns about sexually transmitted diseases, the appropriate tests need to be organized. Women are increasingly demanding hormone tests, erroneously believing that falling androgen levels are to blame. However, an increasing number of publications show no relation between androgen levels and self-reported sexual function.[4]

What is your management plan?

This will depend on what the underlying problem is thought to be.[1,5] She may then wish to have a consultation with her partner present. During this discussion, the following areas can be covered.

Self-help

Sexual materials of all kinds are easy to find: books, DVDs, vibrators, clitoral stimulators, erotic games and lingerie.

Table 30.1 Consensus classification system of female sexual dysfunction

Classification	Definition
I Sexual desire disorders	
A Hypoactive sexual desire disorder	The persistent or recurrent deficiency (or absence) of sexual fantasies/thoughts and/or desire for or receptivity to sexual activity, which causes personal distress
B Sexual aversion disorder	The persistent or recurrent phobic aversion and avoidance of sexual contact with a sexual partner, which causes personal distress
II Sexual arousal disorders	The persistent or recurrent inability to attain or maintain sufficient sexual excitement, causing personal distress, which may be expressed as a lack of subjective excitement, or genital (lubrication/swelling) or other somatic responses
III Orgasmic disorder	The persistent or recurrent difficulty, delay in or absence of attaining orgasm after sufficient sexual stimulation and arousal, which causes personal distress
IV Sexual pain disorders	
A Dyspareunia	The recurrent or persistent genital pain associated with sexual intercourse
B Vaginismus	The recurrent or persistent involuntary spasm of the musculature of the outer third of the vagina, which interferes with vaginal penetration and causes personal distress
C Non-coital sexual pain disorders	Recurrent or persistent genital pain induced by non-coital sexual stimulation

Each of the categories above is subtyped on the basis of the medical history, physical examination and laboratory tests as (A) lifelong versus acquired, (B) generalized versus situational, or (C) aetiology (organic, psychogenic, mixed or unknown).
Source: adapted from Basson *et al.* 2000.[3]

If lubrication is a problem, this may be improved by lubricants and bioadhesive moisturizers. Many different water-based lubricants are now available. Oil-based lubricants, such as peach kernel or sweet almond oils, which last longer than water-based lubricants, have the potential to break down the latex in condoms. This has important implications for the prevention of sexually transmitted diseases. Bioadhesive moisturizers have the advantage that timing of application is not dependent on intercourse.

Psychosexual therapy

Psychosexual therapy (also referred to as sex therapy or psychosexual counselling) has proven success rates. Both partners should be encouraged to attend. Following initial assessment, the therapist will give the couple information about how sexual problems arise and the various treatment options available.

Pharmacotherapy

Androgens

Androgens have been implicated in women's libido but the data are conflicting.[1,4] It is important to remember that other aspects of relationship issues are crucial and complete reliance on androgen treatments is likely to result in poor outcomes.

Testosterone

Several studies have shown a benefit of testosterone therapy in post-menopausal women, but mainly in those using oestrogen.[6] In the United Kingdom, the only licensed preparation for women for many years was subcutaneous implants. Patches for female use are now available. There seems to be no increase in risk in either breast cancer or endometrial hyperplasia from the addition of androgen therapy but data are limited and conflicting.[7,8]

Tibolone

Tibolone is a synthetic steroid compound which is itself inert, but which on absorption is converted *in vivo* to metabolites with oestrogenic, progestogenic and androgenic actions. In post-menopausal woman, tibolone has a positive effect on the vagina, mood, menopausal symptoms, bone and sexual well-being but without stimulation of the breast or endometrium. A number of studies have found tibolone to enhance sexual function.[9]

Dehydroepiandrosterone

Dehydroepiandrosterone (DHEA) and its sulphated form DHEA-S, the androgen precursors made in the adrenal glands, are converted to testosterone. DHEA is not a licensed treatment. Only one double-blind, placebo-controlled, crossover study of DHEA over a four-month period has been done, and this was in women with adrenal insufficiency and low DHEA.[9] The study found that DHEA improved well-being and sexuality but safety is uncertain.

Oestrogens

Low-dose vaginal oestrogens are effective treatments for vaginal dryness and dyspareunia. The options available are low-dose natural oestrogens such as vaginal oestriol by cream or pessary, or oestradiol by tablet or ring. Long-term treatment is required since symptoms return on cessation of therapy. With the recommended dose regimens no adverse endometrial effects should be incurred, and a progestogen need not be added for endometrial protection with such low-dose preparations.[10]

Recent Developments

 The patient might ask for non-hormonal treatment. The results of trials of sildenafil in women are conflicting. Bupropion is an antidepressant that inhibits reuptake of noradrenaline and dopamine. It may improve sexual function, and increases in ratings for sex drive have been found in placebo-controlled studies.[9] Development of other agents assessed in placebo-controlled trials is awaited.

Conclusion

 Sexual problems in women are common and need to be discussed sensitively as they increase with age. In women aged 57 to 85 years the most prevalent sexual problems among women were low desire (43%), difficulty with vaginal lubrication (39%), and inability to climax (34%).[11] After discussion it is established that she finds intercourse painful and this may be the underlying factor and she decides to try vaginal oestrogens first.

Further Reading

1 Tomlinson JM, Rees M, Mander T (eds). *Sexual Health and the Menopause*. London: Royal Society of Medicine Press and British Menopause Society Publications, 2005.

2 Dennerstein L, Lehert P, Burger H, Guthrie J. Sexuality. *Am J Med* 2005; **118** (12 Suppl 2): 59–63.

3 Basson R, Berman J, Burnett A, Derogatis L, Ferguson D, Fourcroy J, Goldstein I, Graziottin A, Heiman J, Laan E, Leiblum S, Padma-Nathan H, Rosen R, Segraves K, Segraves RT, Shabsigh R, Sipski M, Wagner G, Whipple B. Report of the international consensus development conference on female sexual dysfunction: definitions and classifications. *J Urol* 2000; **163**: 888–93.

4 Davis SR, Davison SL, Donath S, Bell RJ. Circulating androgen levels and self-reported sexual function in women. *JAMA* 2005; **294**: 91–6.

5 Miller HB, Hunt JS. Female sexual dysfunction: review of the disorder and evidence for available treatment alternatives. *J Pharm Pract* 2003; **16**: 200–8.

6 Davis SR, van der Mooren MJ, van Lunsen RH, Lopes P, Ribot C, Rees M, Moufarege A, Rodenberg C, Buch A, Purdie DW. Efficacy and safety of a testosterone patch for the treatment of hypoactive sexual desire disorder in surgically menopausal women: a randomized, placebo-controlled trial. *Menopause* 2006; **13**: 387–96.

7 Tamimi RM, Hankinson SE, Chen WY, Rosner B, Colditz GA. Combined estrogen and testosterone use and risk of breast cancer in postmenopausal women. *Arch Intern Med* 2006; **166**: 1483–9.

8 Dimitrakakis C, Jones RA, Liu A, Bondy CA. Breast cancer incidence in postmenopausal women using testosterone in addition to usual hormone therapy. *Menopause* 2004; **11**: 531–5.

9 Wylie KR. Sexuality and the menopause. *J Br Menopause Soc* 2006; **12**: 149–52.

10 Rees M, Purdie DW (eds). *Management of the Menopause: The Handbook*. London: Royal Society of Medicine Press, 2006.

11 Lindau ST, Schumm LP, Laumann EO, Levinson W, O'Muircheartaigh CA, Waite LJ. A study of sexuality and health among older adults in the United States. *N Engl J Med* 2007; **357**: 762–4.

31 Dyspareunia

Case History

A 28-year-old woman attends, complaining of pain on intercourse. She is in a new relationship and is taking the combined oral contraceptive pill.

Is this superficial or deep dyspareunia?

What are the possible causes?

How would you reach a diagnosis?

How would you approach the management of each condition?

Background

Dyspareunia is recurrent or persistent genital pain associated with sexual intercourse. It may be classified as primary, when pain has always been present on sexual intercourse, or secondary, when intercourse has in the past been pain-free. It may also be classified as 'superficial' or 'deep', depending on the site of the pain.

Superficial dyspareunia

Discomfort is usually introital and less commonly mid-vaginal. The cause may be poor arousal and/or lubrication, or topical irritants such as spermicides or latex. A number of vulval conditions may also cause discomfort.

Infection resulting in vulvitis/vulvovaginitis, such as Candida or genital herpes, can be a cause of superficial dyspareunia.

Vulvar vestibulitis (also known as focal vulvitis/vestibulitis) is a clinical diagnosis and the aetiology is unknown.[1] It is characterized by pain at the introitus, on penetration during sexual intercourse or on the insertion of tampons. There is often a long history. On examination there is focal tenderness at the vestibule with variable erythema. General advice on vulval care should be given, including the avoidance of soap, shampoo and other potential irritants. Emollient creams and ointments may be used as a substitute. Tight-fitting garments may irritate the area and spermicidally lubricated condoms should be avoided.

Many specific treatments for vulvar vestibulitis exist; however, there is a lack of well-designed clinical trials. The natural history is that remission can occur in up to 50% of patients.[1] Topical local anaesthetics may relieve pain during sexual intercourse. Pain modifiers, such as amitriptyline in small doses, have been used; other approaches include topical steroids, behavioural therapy and, as a last resort, surgery.[2]

Vulvodynia (dysaesthetic vulvodynia) is also of unknown aetiology and diagnosis is once again clinical.[1] Pain is felt over a much broader area and can extend perianally or to the upper thighs. It is more prevalent in peri- or post-menopausal women and there is often a long history. The vulva appears normal, with tenderness to light touch over the labia.

General advice on vulval care should, once again, be given. Amitriptyline and gabapentin have been used with some success[3] and selective serotonin reuptake inhibitors (SSRIs) may also be effective. Local anaesthetics are not generally helpful as they only provide short-term relief.

Vulval dermatitis may follow infection or be irritant, allergic, atopic or seborrhoeic. Itching and soreness are usually presenting features and there may be erythema, lichenification and fissuring of the vulval skin. Dermatological referral may be necessary, but most cases can be treated with topical steroids.

Vulval lichen sclerosus is an inflammatory condition of unknown aetiology, although genetic predisposition, infections and autoimmune factors have all been implicated in its pathogenesis.[4] Symptoms include irritation, soreness and urinary symptoms. The skin may appear pale and atrophic or there may be erosions, blistering, purpura, fissuring and hyperkeratosis. A biopsy may be necessary to confirm the diagnosis, and treatment is usually with potent topical steroids. Follow-up is essential due to the potential risk of malignant change.[4]

Vulval intraepithelial neoplasia is a rare, but important condition to exclude in older patients.

Deep dyspareunia

The discomfort is felt on deep penetration and may be due to lack of arousal, but more often is related to pelvic pathology. Several of the conditions mentioned below are covered in more detail in separate chapters.

Pelvic inflammatory disease is caused by spread of infection from the lower to the upper genital tract, most commonly due to *Chlamydia trachomatis*. As well as deep dyspareunia there may be vaginal discharge or bleeding, dysuria, pelvic pain and pyrexia. Diagnosis is clinical and confirmed by the presence of cervical motion tenderness and/or adnexal tenderness. A sexual health screen should be carried out and treatment involves antibiotics to cover *Chlamydia trachomatis*, *Neisseria gonorrhoea* and anaerobes.

Endometriosis is the presence of ectopic uterine endometrial tissue outside the uterine cavity and musculature. This ectopic endometrium responds to hormonal changes during the menstrual cycle, with subsequent bleeding, inflammation and, if the ovaries are affected, the development of endometriotic ovarian cysts.[6] Exact prevalence is difficult to predict accurately but is likely to be in excess of 33% of women presenting with chronic pelvic pain.[7] Endometriosis is uncommon in post-menopausal women as it is oestrogen dependent. Symptoms also include cyclical or chronic pelvic pain, secondary dysmenorrhoea and menorrhagia.

Diagnosis of endometriosis is confirmed on laparoscopy, and treatment depends upon extent, symptoms, age and fertility plans, as endometriosis is also associated with subfertility.[8] Specialist referral is usually advised.

Gynaecological, pelvic or abdominal surgery or radiotherapy may cause deep dyspareunia, usually as a result of pelvic adhesions. **Genital or pelvic tumours**, including fibroids, may also cause deep dyspareunia.

Irritable bowel syndrome may sometimes present with deep dyspareunia, in the absence of any other gynaecological symptoms. **Positional dyspareunia** should also be considered, particularly if all other investigations are normal. Sometimes deep thrusting can cause pressure on the ovary, producing pain.

Vaginismus should be mentioned as it may present with dypareunia, but in the Diagnostic and Statistical Manual of Mental Disorders – Fourth Edition (DSM-IV) it is considered to be a separate disorder in the subcategory of sexual dysfunctions.

Vaginismus is recurrent or persistent involuntary spasm of the musculature of the outer third of the vagina[9] and can be primary or secondary. It may develop as part of a conditioning response to adverse physical and/or psychological stimuli. It may in fact develop as a result of dyspareunia due to another cause. Attempted penetration results in pain and is often impossible. Treatment should ideally be multidisciplinary, with psychological input, education and graded vaginal dilatation, with or without the use of vaginal trainers. Vaginismus is covered more extensively in Case 33: Vaginismus.

Recent Developments

Surgery for vulvar vestibulitis was first described in 1981 and is generally considered to be a last resort. However studies of complete vulvar vestibulectomy with vaginal advancement appears to have good results with a 93% satisfaction rate at 26 months.[10] However, such a radical approach should only be undertaken in specialist centres.

Conclusion

Dyspareunia is a very sensitive issue. It is essential, when considering the diagnosis for a woman presenting with dyspareunia, also to consider psychosexual influences. Comorbidity with other sexual dysfunctions, such as loss of libido, orgasmic difficulties and arousal disorders, is not uncommon in patients with chronic dyspareunia.

Further Reading

1 Edwards S, Handfield-Jones S, Gull S. National guideline on the management of vulval conditions. *Int J STD AIDS* 2002; **13**: 411–15.

2 Goldstein A. Surgical techniques: Surgery for Vulvar Vestibulitis syndrome. *J Sex Med* 2006; **3**: 559–62.

3 Smart OC, MacLean AB. Vulvodynia. *Curr Opin Obstet Gynecol* 2003; **15**: 497–500.

4 Yesudian PD, Sugunendran H, Bates CM, O'Mahony C. Lichen sclerosus. *Int J STD AIDS* 2005; **16**: 465–73.

5 Butcher J. Female sexual problems II: sexual pain and sexual fears. In: Tomlinson J (ed). *ABC of Sexual Health*, 2nd edn. Oxford: Blackwell Publishing, 2005; 25–8.

6 Prodigy Guidance 2006. Endometriosis. www.cks.library.nhs.uk/endometriosis (accessed 17 09 07)

7 Guo SW, Wang Y. The prevalence of endometriosis in women with chronic pelvic pain. *Gynecol Obstet Invest* 2006; **62**: 121–30.

8 Farquhar C. Endometriosis. *BMJ* 2007; **334**: 249–53.

9 Crowley T, Richardson D, Goldmeier D. Recommendations for the management of vaginismus: BASHH Special Interest Group for Sexual Dysfunction. *Int J STD AIDS* 2006; **17**: 14–18.

10 Goldstein AT, Klingman D, Christopher K, Johnson C, Marinoff SC. Surgical treatment of vulvar vestibulitis syndrome: outcome assessment derived from a postoperative questionnaire. *J Sex Med* 2006; **3**: 923–31.

32 Vaginal Discharge

Case History

A 28-year-old woman presents with a six-week history of an offensive vaginal discharge. She is sexually active and takes the combined oral contraceptive (COC) pill.

What are the important aspects of the history?

What is the differential diagnosis?

What are the treatment options?

Background

Vaginal discharge is a common presenting symptom and there are a range of possible diagnoses. Causes may broadly be divided into physiological and pathological.

Physiological discharge

Lactobacilli form the normal vaginal flora and colonize the vaginal epithelium. They maintain a vaginal pH of 3.8–4.4 and play a role in the defence against infection. Normal vaginal discharge is altered by a number of factors such as hormonal changes as part of the menstrual cycle, pregnancy and hormonal contraception. Physiological discharge is usually clear or white and odourless.

Pathological discharge

Infection

Infections causing an alteration in vaginal discharge may or may not be sexually transmitted (Figure 32.1). Sexually transmitted infections are dealt with in more detail in Case 35: Sexually Transmitted Infections, and would include *Trichomonas vaginalis*, *Neisseria gonorrhoea* and *Chlamydia trachomatis*. Ulceration from *Herpes simplex* may also result in a vaginal discharge.

   Bacterial vaginosis (BV) is a common cause of vaginal discharge and results from a change in bacterial flora of the vagina from mainly lactobacilli to high concentrations of anaerobic bacteria. The main bacterium found in BV is *Gardnerella vaginalis*, although this can be found on culture in approximately 50% of healthy, asymptomatic women.[1] Replacement of lactobacilli leads to an increase in vaginal pH to as high as pH 7. Although BV is not regarded as a sexually transmitted infection, it is more common in sexually active than non-sexually active women. It is also more prevalent in black women than white, those with an intrauterine contraceptive device and those who smoke.[2]

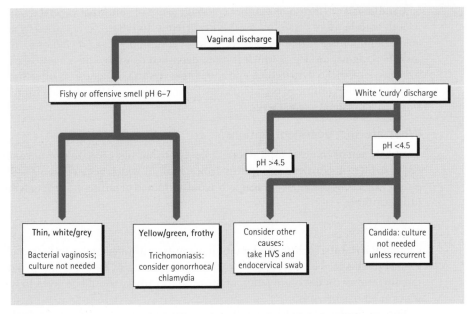

Figure 32.1 Diagnosis of candida and bacterial vaginosis. HVS, high vaginal swab. *Source*: Smellie *et al.* 2006.[8]

What are the important aspects of the history?

The main complaint is of an offensive, fishy-smelling discharge, usually in the absence of pain or irritation. On speculum examination there is usually evidence of a thin white or grey homogeneous discharge.

What is the differential diagnosis?

Several diagnostic tests exist and a high vaginal swab should be taken from the posterior fornix. Application of the **Amsel criteria**[3] is the gold standard but is not always available in practice. At least three of the four criteria must be present for a diagnosis to be confirmed:

1 Thin, white homogeneous discharge

2 Clue cells on microscopy of wet mount

3 pH of vaginal fluid >4.5

4 Release of a fishy odour on adding alkali (10% potassium hydroxide)

An alternative is to use a Gram-stained vaginal smear, with the **Hay/Ison criteria**[4] or the **Nugent score**.[5]

Complications of BV are rare, except in pregnancy or following termination of pregnancy, and symptoms may resolve spontaneously. The antibiotic treatment of choice is oral metronidazole 400 mg twice daily for 5–7 days, or as a single oral dose of 2 g if compliance is an issue. Alternative treatment regimes include intravaginal metronidazole gel or intravaginal clindamycin cream. Advice should be given to avoid vaginal douching and the use of perfumed or antiseptic products during washing.

Candidiasis or 'thrush' is another common cause of abnormal vaginal discharge and is dealt with in more detail in Case 34: Recurrent Candidiasis. It is caused by abnormal colonization of the vagina by yeast cells, most commonly *Candida albicans*. Symptoms include a vaginal discharge which is often described as white and 'cheese-like', itching, soreness, superficial dyspareunia and sometimes dysuria. Diagnosis is often made clinically but may be confirmed on microscopy from a high vaginal swab taken from the anterior fornix or lateral vaginal walls.

What are the treatment options?

The treatment of choice is topical imidazoles (clotrimazole, econazole or miconazole) or oral triazoles (fluconazole and itraconazole), both of which achieve an 80%–95% cure rate.[6,7] Advice should be given, again, to avoid perfumed or antiseptic products and tight-fitting clothing.

Other causes

Chemical irritants, such as deodorants, lubricants or disinfectants, can cause a change in vaginal discharge. The discharge is usually accompanied by soreness and irritation and rapidly resolves on discontinuation of the product. Advice should be given to wash with water or emollients only.

Foreign body. Examples include a retained tampon, condom or vaginal sponge. Examination to exclude the presence of a foreign body is essential, and after removal the possibility of secondary infection should be considered.

Cervical ectropion may cause a clear, mucoid discharge with or without post-coital bleeding. The presence of an ectropion can be confirmed on speculum examination and, if severe, referral for local treatment may be considered.

Endocervical polyp may be present and may also cause abnormal bleeding. Speculum examination should confirm the diagnosis and removal of the polyp for histological examination should be carried out.

Tumours of the vulva, vagina, cervix or endometrium should always be considered in older patients and appropriate investigations carried out.

Post-menopausal atrophic vaginitis may cause a vaginal discharge and is easily confirmed on clinical examination. Treatment is with topical oestrogen.

Surgery. It is also worth remembering that vaginal discharge may be present for up to six weeks following surgery of the vagina or uterus.

Less common causes of vaginal discharge may include physical trauma, or vesicovaginal or rectovaginal fistulae.

Recent Developments

Vaginal discharge is one of the most common conditions for which women seek medical care. Of concern is that women with vaginal complaints may self-treat incorrectly with over-the-counter drugs. It is essential that there is ease of consultation for this problem and that health professionals undertake the appropriate investigations and recommend effective treatments.

Conclusion

Most cases of vaginal discharge can be diagnosed from a relevant history, clinical examination and appropriate investigation. Treatment should be given for pathological causes but often simple reassurance and advice is all that is required.

Further Reading

1   CKS Guidance 2006. Bacterial vaginosis. www.cks.library.nhs.uk/bacterial_vaginosis (accessed 17 09 07)

2   Clinical Effectiveness Group (Association for Genitourinary Medicine and the Medical Society for the Study of Venereal Diseases). National guideline for the management of bacterial vaginosis (2006). www.bashh.org/guidelines/2006/bv_final_0706.pdf (accessed 17 09 07)

3   Amsel R, Totten PA, Spiegel CA, Chen KC, Eschenbach D, Holmes KK. Nonspecific vaginitis. Diagnostic criteria and microbial and epidemiologic associations. *Am J Med* 1983; **74**: 14–22.

4   Ison CA, Hay PE. Validation of a simplified grading of Gram stained vaginal smears for use in genitourinary medicine clinics. *Sex Transm Infect* 2002; **78**: 413–15.

5   Nugent RP, Krohn MA, Hillier SL. Reliability of diagnosing bacterial vaginosis is improved by a standardized method of gram stain interpretation. *J Clin Microbiol* 1991; **29**: 297–301.

6   Clinical Effectiveness Group (Association for Genitourinary Medicine and the Medical Society for the Study of Venereal Diseases). National guideline on the management of vulvovaginal candidiasis (2002). www.bashh.org/guidelines/2002/candida_0601.pdf (accessed 17 09 07)

7   CKS Guidance 2005. Candida – female genital. www.cks.library.nhs.uk/candida_female_genital (accessed 17 09 07)

8   Smellie WS, Forth J, Sundar S, Kalu E, McNulty CA, Sherriff E, Watson ID, Croucher C, Reynolds TM, Carey PJ. Best practice in primary care pathology: review 4. *J Clin Pathol* 2006; **59**: 893–902.

PROBLEM

33 Vaginismus

Case History

A 23-year-old woman presents with the inability to have intercourse. She had no problems with her first partner when she was 16 years old, although this relationship ended six months later. Because she was sexually active her general practitioner performed a cervical smear for her when she was 17 years old. She found this excruciatingly painful. It was suggested that the pain was due to a retroverted uterus and she has not attended for a smear since, despite numerous reminders. She has been unable to have intercourse with two partners subsequently, despite feeling aroused, and is concerned that her current relationship will end.

What physical conditions need to be considered before a diagnosis of vaginismus can be made?

What factors are associated with vaginismus?

What are the aims of treatment?

How are these aims achieved?

Background

The term 'vaginismus' was first used in the nineteenth century[1] and is now thought to be one of the commonest female sexual problems. The true prevalence is unknown; however, it is identified in 10%–20% of women requesting help for sexual dysfunction.[2] Definitions vary as to whether or not spasm of the muscles surrounding the lower third of the vagina is included or whether it is difficulty in allowing vaginal entry, often associated with involuntary pelvic muscle contraction.[3] Although it occurs when the woman anticipates intercourse, there is often fear of any object being placed in the vagina, thus tampons are not used and gynaecological examinations are not well tolerated. The condition may be primary, where non-painful penetrative intercourse has never occurred, or secondary, where previously the woman has experienced non-painful penetrative vaginal intercourse.[3]

What physical conditions need to be considered before a diagnosis of vaginismus can be made?

Vaginismus is thought to occur as a conditioned response secondary to adverse physical or psychological stimuli. Thus, any pathology which causes dyspareunia, either superficial or deep, can set up a cycle whereby fear of pain causes involuntary spasm which causes further pain, reinforcing the conditioned response (Figure 33.1).[4] Specific conditions which should be looked for and excluded are shown in Table 33.1.

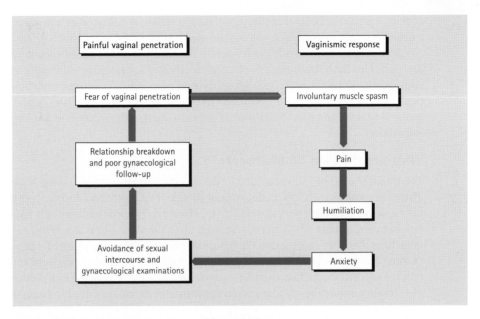

Figure 33.1 Cycle of vaginismus. *Source*: Butcher 2005.[4]

Table 33.1 Causes of dyspareunia	
Cause	Example
Infections	Herpes simplex
	Pelvic inflammatory disease
	Chronic cervicitis
	Chronic urethritis
Atrophic vaginitis	
Lichen sclerosus	
Vulval dysaesthesia	
Endometriosis	
Trauma	Episiotomy
	Tear

What factors are associated with vaginismus?

Early traumatic experiences are thought to predispose to vaginismus. Thus, traumatic sexual experiences, unsympathetic gynaecological examinations and assault are all associated factors.[3] However, it has also been reported that, unlike women who report chronic pelvic pain, vaginismus is not usually associated with a history of abuse (physical or sexual).[5] A background of religious orthodoxy has also been associated with the condition,[6] possibly because of feelings of guilt about the experience, or because inadequate information had been given about sexual experiences and concerns about long-term damage are therefore able to arise. False beliefs (known as psychosexual fantasies) often coexist, such as the belief that the vagina is too small to accommodate a penis or that it is a delicate, fragile organ which will be damaged during intercourse.[3] Such beliefs can arise as a result of comments made inadvertently, for example at the time of episiotomy repair, and clinicians should therefore think carefully about what is said at vulnerable times. As a consequence of vaginismus, male sexual dysfunction such as impotence; relationship difficulties or breakdowns; and alterations in psychological profile such as depression and low self-esteem can arise.[7] 'Vaginismus' may also be the presentation of a male partner's impotence.

What are the aims of treatment?

Treatment should be individualized to the specific woman/couple and her/their desires. Thus, for most women, successful vaginal penetrative intercourse and an improved sexual experience for both partners is the aim. However, in some instances the woman may not feel comfortable with intercourse even after the vaginismus has resolved. Current guidelines therefore suggest that the basis of treatment should be to enable the woman to become more comfortable with her genitals, followed by graded exposure to different types of vaginal penetration in order to overcome her fear of penetration.[3] For some couples, fertility is the ultimate aim and an appropriate referral may need to be made.

How are these aims achieved?

A number of different approaches are described, one of which is a combination of behavioural and desensitization exercises using relaxation and graded vaginal trainers. Education is also important and there may be a need for exploration of fantasies before they can be dispelled.[3] Hypnotherapy,[7] physiotherapy using biofeedback, amitriptyline and local injections with botulinum toxin[8] have all been reported to have good results. Cognitive behavioural therapy (CBT) may be of help.[9] If physical causes have been excluded, CBT is usually highly successful, with some authors reporting up to 100% success.

Recent Developments

A novel approach is the use of topical application of lignocaine gel along with systematic desensitization resulting in successful consummation. However this is currently limited to a case report.[10]

Conclusion

The woman should feel that she is in control at all times during treatment, and specific requests about the gender of the doctor or presence or absence of a chaperone should be complied with if at all possible. To what extent her partner is involved should also be her decision, although involvement should be encouraged.

Further Reading

1 Sims MJ. On vaginismus. *Trans Obstet Soc London* 1861; **3**: 356–67.

2 Schnyder U, Schnyder-Lüthi C, Balinari P, Blaser A. Therapy for vaginismus: in vivo versus in vitro desensitization. *Can J Psychiatry* 1998; **43**: 941–4.

3 Crowley T, Richardson D, Goldmeier D. Recommendations for the management of vaginismus: BASHH Special Interest Group for Sexual Dysfunction. *Int J STD AIDS* 2006; **17**: 14–18.

4 Butcher J. Female sexual problems II: sexual pain and sexual fears. In: Tomlinson J (ed). *ABC of Sexual Health*, 2nd edn. Oxford: Blackwell Publishing, 2005; 25–8.

5 Meana M, Binik YM, Khalife S, Cohen DR. Biopsychosocial profile of women with dyspareunia. *Obstet Gynecol* 1997; **90**: 583–9.

6 Stanley E. Vaginismus. *Br Med J (Clin Res Ed)* 1981; **282**: 1435–7.

7 Al-Sughayir MA. Vaginismus treatment. Hypnotherapy versus behavior therapy. *Neurosciences* 2005; **10**: 163–7.

8 Ghazizadeh S, Nikzad M. Botulinum toxin in the treatment of refractory vaginismus. *Obstet Gynecol* 2004; **104**: 922–5.

9 ter Kuile MM, van Lankveld JJ, de Groot E, Melles R, Neffs J, Zandbergen M. Cognitive-behavioral therapy for women with lifelong vaginismus: process and prognostic factors. *Behav Res Ther* 2007; **45**: 359–73.

10 Praharaj SK, Verma P, Arora M. Topical lignocaine for vaginismus: a case report. *Int J Impot Res* 2006; **18**: 568–9.

Urogenital problems

PROBLEM

34 Recurrent Candidiasis

Case History

A 25-year-old woman comes complaining of a vaginal discharge, itching and soreness. From the history, a diagnosis of vulvovaginal candidiasis (VVC), otherwise referred to as vaginal thrush, is likely. She has been using a cream that she obtained from the chemist with some relief, but reports that she has similar symptoms every few months.

How would you confirm a diagnosis of VVC?

What is the differential diagnosis?

What are potential precipitating factors?

What are the treatment options?

Background

VVC is the second most common cause of vaginitis and vaginal discharge after bacterial vaginosis and is characterized by abnormal colonization of the vagina by yeast cells. The lifetime incidence of VVC is estimated to be between 50% and 75%.[1]

The commonest causative agent is *Candida albicans*, accounting for 80%–95% of infections, and *Candida glabrata* is responsible for a further 5%.[1] Other yeast infections are less common and are generally more difficult to treat. Candida is often present in the vagina of asymptomatic women and becomes pathological following a change in the vaginal environment. Infection may be classified as 'acute' or 'recurrent'. Recurrent candidiasis is defined as four or more episodes over the period of a year and occurs in less than 5% of women of reproductive age.[2]

How would you confirm a diagnosis of VVC?

Diagnosis may be clinical or confirmed by laboratory testing. Typical symptoms include a vaginal discharge, itching, soreness, superficial dyspareunia and sometimes dysuria. Signs may include a non-offensive vaginal discharge, vulval and vaginal erythema, fissuring, oedema and the presence of satellite lesions.

If a diagnosis cannot be reached on clinical grounds alone, or symptoms become recurrent, a high vaginal swab may be taken from the anterior fornix or lateral vaginal walls. Microscopy looking for spores and/or pseudohyphae detects up to 70% of cases,[1] and culture is helpful to exclude other diagnoses or for identification of resistant species.

What is the differential diagnosis?

Differential diagnosis includes bacterial vaginosis, sexually transmitted infections (such as trichomoniasis, gonorrhoea, herpes, chlamydia), normal physiological discharge, local irritants, skin conditions (eczema, psoriasis), atrophic vaginitis (in post-menopausal women), foreign body (such as a retained tampon) and, rarely, malignancy (see Case 32: Vaginal Discharge). Clearly, individual symptoms and signs will vary.

What are potential precipitating factors?

VVC is more common in women of reproductive age as *Candida albicans* flourishes in an oestrogen-rich environment. For this reason, it is also more common in pregnancy.

Controversy exists regarding the significance of certain forms of contraception in relation to recurrent VVC. There is no good evidence of an association with the oral contraceptive pill; condoms probably do not cause VVC *per se*, but certain spermicides may increase the likelihood of infection by harming the natural vaginal flora; and there is some evidence of an association of VVC with intrauterine devices.[2] VVC is not a sexually transmitted infection but some studies report an increased incidence with certain sexual practices, notably oral sex.[3]

Diabetes mellitus increases the incidence of VVC and cases are more likely in patients with poor diabetic control.[4] Certain drugs, such as immunosuppressives and broad-spectrum antibiotics, also increase the frequency of VVC. The incidence of VVC in human immunodeficiency virus (HIV)-infected women is unknown.[5] Vaginal Candida colonization rates among HIV-infected women are higher than those for seronegative women with similar demographic characteristics and high-risk behaviours; colonization rates correlate with increasing severity of immunosuppression. Symptomatic VVC is more frequent in seropositive women and similarly correlates with severity of immunodeficiency.

Candida tends to thrive in warm environments, so advice is generally given to avoid tight-fitting clothing and to wear cotton underwear and skirts rather than trousers. Evidence for this is conflicting. Equally, feminine hygiene may have some impact, sanitary towels possibly increasing the incidence of VVC.[6,7]

Depletion of lactobacilli has been implicated in the pathogenesis of VVC, leading to the popularity of oral and vaginal delivery of live cultures of lactobacilli. However, use of these preparations is not at present recommended due to lack of evidence of efficacy.[1]

What are the treatment options?

VVC can be a distressing problem, particularly if recurrent, and can lead to possible psychosexual problems and depression. Patients should be treated sensitively and given a full explanation of the condition. Preventative measures, such as avoidance of irritants and synthetic underwear, should be discussed and reassurance should be given that VVC is not a sexually transmitted infection.

First episodes of VVC may be diagnosed clinically but swabs may be required if there is doubt about the diagnosis, symptoms are recurrent or there has been no response to treatment. Treatment may begin while waiting for swab results.

Topical imidazoles (clotrimazole, econazole or miconazole) are an effective cure for uncomplicated VVC.[1] Effectiveness of topical treatments is related to dose rather than length of treatment[5,8,9] and intravaginal application as well as external topical application is required for treatment to be effective. Oral triazoles (fluconazole and itraconazole) have also been shown to be effective in the treatment of VVC. Topical and oral azole therapies give an 80%–95% clinical and mycological cure rate in non-pregnant women.[2]

Other drug treatments include topical nystatin, oral ketoconazole and topical povidone-iodine. Topical nystatin is more effective against certain resistant yeast strains such as *Candida glabrata* and may therefore be useful in treatment failure, but it is taken as a 14-day course of treatment and may stain clothes yellow so is not used as a first-line option. Oral ketoconazole has been linked to fulminant hepatitis and is therefore only rarely used in treating recurrent VVC that is unresponsive to other treatments. Povidone-iodine is an antiseptic available in topical intravaginal formulations and is licensed for use in non-specific vaginal infections.[10] However, there is little evidence of its efficacy in the treatment of VVC.

Symptomatic and asymptomatic VVC is more common in pregnancy and topical azole treatment is recommended. Oral therapy is contraindicated. Treatment courses may need to be extended in these patients. Women who are immunocompromised, either by medication (long-term corticosteroids or other immunosuppressive drugs) or illness (such as HIV infection), often also require longer courses.

VVC is not sexually transmitted and there is no evidence that treating the male partner is of any benefit.[5,6]

Treatment regimens for recurrent VVC are empirical and not based on randomized controlled trials. They usually involve an induction period consisting of 6–12 days of daily treatment with a topical imidazole followed by a maintenance regime for six months. Typical regimens include fluconazole 100 mg weekly or clotrimazole pessaries 500 mg weekly. The use of antifungal drugs in maintenance therapy is not licensed and relapse on cessation may occur in at least 50% of cases.[2] These women may require even longer courses of maintenance therapy following relapse.

Treatment failure in uncomplicated VVC is unusual and it is worth considering factors such as poor compliance, incorrect diagnosis, irritants, mixed infection or an underlying cause, such as diabetes.

Recent Developments

1   Based on available data, therapy for VVC in HIV-infected women should not differ from that for seronegative women.[5] Although long-term prophylactic therapy with fluconazole at a dose of 200 mg weekly has been effective in reducing *C. albicans* colonization and symptomatic VVC, this regimen is not recommended for routine primary prophylaxis in HIV-infected women in the absence of recurrent VVC.

2   Depletion of lactobacilli has been implicated in the pathogenesis of vulvovaginal candidiasis which has led to studies of live cultures of lactobacilli administered either orally or intravaginally.[1] However, the evidence is poor and there is no regulatory authority regarding the contents of these products. Other products sometimes used in the prevention of vulvovaginal candidiasis include pH reducing agents and oils, but there is no documented evidence to support their use. Tampons impregnated with tea tree oil are used by some women, but again there is no evidence of efficacy. In addition, it should be remembered that these products can provoke allergic reaction.

Conclusion

Since this patient has had several episodes, it is likely that she will need long-term treatment with a maintenance regime for 6 months.

Further Reading

1   CKS Guidance 2005. Candida – female genital. www.cks.library.nhs.uk/candida_female_genital (accessed 17 09 07)

2   Clinical Effectiveness Group (Association for Genitourinary Medicine and the Medical Society for the Study of Venereal Diseases). National guideline on the management of vulvovaginal candidiasis (2002). www.bashh.org/guidelines/2002/candida_0601.pdf (accessed 17 09 07)

3   Reed BD, Gorenflo DW, Gillespie BW, Pierson CL, Zazove P. Sexual behaviors and other risk factors for Candida vulvovaginitis. *J Womens Health Gend Based Med* 2000; **9**: 645–55.

4   de Leon EM, Jacober SJ, Sobel JD, Foxman B. Prevalence and risk factors for vaginal Candida colonization in women with type 1 and type 2 diabetes. *BMC Infect Dis* 2002; **2**: 1.

5   Centers for Disease Control and Prevention. Sexually Transmitted Diseases Treatment Guidelines 2006. Diseases characterized by vaginal discharge. www.cdc.gov/std/treatment/2006/vaginal-discharge.htm (accessed 17 09 07)

6   Mardh PA, Rodrigues AG, Genc M, Novikova N, Martinez-de-Oliveira J, Guaschino S. Facts and myths on recurrent vulvovaginal candidosis – a review on epidemiology, clinical manifestations, diagnosis, pathogenesis and therapy. *Int J STD AIDS* 2002; **13**: 522–39.

7   Patel DA, Gillespie B, Sobel JD, Leaman D, Nyirjesy P, Weitz MV, Foxman B. Risk factors for recurrent vulvovaginal candidiasis in women receiving maintenance antifungal therapy: results of a prospective cohort study. *Am J Obstet Gynecol* 2004; **190**: 644–53.

8 Sobel JD. Management of patients with recurrent vulvovaginal candidiasis. *Drugs* 2003; **63**: 1059–66.

9 Sobel JD. Management of recurrent vulvovaginal candidiasis: unresolved issues. *Curr Infect Dis Rep* 2006; **8**: 481–6.

10 British Medical Association and the Royal Pharmaceutical Society of Great Britain. *British National Formulary*, Vol. 53. March 2007 edition.

PROBLEM

35 Sexually Transmitted Infections

Case History

A 23-year-old woman visits the clinic requesting a 'check-up'. She had unprotected sex with a casual partner three weeks ago and now has some offensive vaginal discharge. She has recently begun a new relationship and is concerned about the possibility of infection.

What are the important questions to ask as part of a sexual history?

What is the differential diagnosis and which tests should be undertaken?

Background

Sexually transmitted infections (STIs) remain a major public health challenge. In the United States (US), the Center for Disease Control and Prevention estimate that 19 million new infections occur each year, almost half of them among young people aged 15 to 24 years.[1] Direct medical costs associated with STIs in the US are estimated at up to $14.1 billion annually. In the United Kingdom (UK) there has been a gradual rise in the number of diagnoses of acute STIs.[2] Chlamydia cases increased by 206% between 1996 and 2005, gonorrhoea by 55% and syphilis, although uncommon, by 1949%. In 2001, the UK Department of Health produced *The national strategy for sexual health and HIV*.[3] The key objectives are to ensure that all individuals have access to the knowledge and skills necessary to achieve positive sexual health and that services should be available to all who require them.[4] Specifically, the aims are to reduce the undiagnosed prevalence and transmission of STIs and human immunodeficiency virus (HIV), to reduce unintended pregnancies and to improve social and health care for people with HIV. Targets were introduced to reduce the incidence of HIV and gonorrhoea by 2007.

What are the important questions to ask as part of a sexual history?

When taking a sexual history, it is important to communicate with the patient on their level and in a non-judgemental manner, assuring confidentiality (Table 35.1). Firstly, details of the presenting complaint should be taken. A description of the discharge, duration of symptoms and the presence of any associated symptoms, such as dyspareunia or dysuria, should be recorded.

Full details of past and present sexual partners, at least for the previous twelve months, should be taken, including use of barrier contraception, whether regular or casual relationships and nationality.

Method of contraception, if any, is important to assess risk of pregnancy and to discuss and provide emergency contraception if appropriate. Previous STI diagnoses and treatment and also confirmation of partner treatment and compliance should be noted.

Details of the last menstrual period and any menstrual irregularities, such as intermenstrual or post-coital bleeding, may give clues to the diagnosis. Finally, as always, a brief medical and drug history should be taken and details of the most recent cervical smear.

Risk factors for STIs include young age, single status, at least two partners in the preceding six months, non-barrier contraception and deprivation.

Table 35.1 Taking a sexual history
Description of discharge
Duration of symptoms
Associated symptoms (e.g. dyspareunia, dysuria)
Details of past and present sexual partners within past twelve months
Method of contraception
Menstrual history
Medical and drug history
Result of most recent cervical smear

What is the differential diagnosis and which tests should be undertaken?

A brief overview of the most common STIs is given below (Table 35.2). When considering one diagnosis, a general screen should always be carried out, with the suspicion of the presence of multiple infection.

Chlamydia is the most common sexually transmitted bacterial infection in the UK and is caused by the obligate intracellular bacterium *Chlamydia trachomatis*. It is asymptomatic in up to 80% of affected women.[5] It is the commonest cause of pelvic inflammatory disease (PID) and accounts for an estimated 43% of ectopic pregnancies.[5]

If symptoms are present, the commonest include post-coital or intermenstrual bleeding, pelvic pain, dysuria, purulent vaginal discharge, mucopurulent cervicitis and/or contact bleeding. Vaginal examination is often unremarkable but if the patient is symptomatic, there may be a discharge or signs of PID.

Table 35.2 A brief overview of common STIs

	Chlamydia	Gonorrhoea	Genital herpes	Trichomoniasis
Symptoms	Asymptomatic in 80%	Vaginal discharge ± lower abdominal pain, dysuria	Painful genital ulceration ± dysuria, vaginal/ urethral discharge, urinary retention	Offensive vaginal discharge but may be absent in 50%
Treatment	Azithromycin, doxycycline	Dependent on local patterns of resistance	Aciclovir, valaciclovir or famciclovir	Metronidazole

An endocervical swab taken to confirm the diagnosis should be inserted into the cervical os and firmly rotated against the endocervix after excess cervical secretions have been removed. The most sensitive (90%–95%) laboratory test is by nucleic acid amplification technique (NAAT) and the detection rate increases with the number of sites sampled. If vaginal examination is not indicated, self-testing can be carried out using a vulvovaginal swab or first-void urine, again using NAAT.

First-line treatment in non-pregnant women is with azithromycin or doxycycline. Ofloxacin is an alternative. Pregnant women should be treated with erythromycin or amoxicillin, with a test of cure.

Gonorrhoea results from infection with the Gram-negative diplococcus *Neisseria gonorrhoeae*. Transmission is by direct spread from one mucous membrane to another, principally the urethra, endocervix, rectum, pharynx and conjunctiva. An increased or altered vaginal discharge is the commonest symptom (in up to 50% of cases); lower abdominal pain and dysuria may also be present.[6] On examination there may be pelvic tenderness, a mucopurulent endocervical discharge and endocervical contact bleeding. Diagnosis is by culture from infected sites, and if a diagnosis of gonorrhoea is suspected, swabs should be taken from the endocervix, urethra, rectum and oropharynx.

Untreated, gonorrhoea may go on to cause PID. Antibiotic treatment is dependent upon local patterns of resistance and advice should always be sought from the local genitourinary service.

Genital herpes is caused by infection with the herpes simplex virus (HSV), a double-stranded DNA virus in the same family as varicella-zoster, cytomegalovirus and Epstein Barr.[7] The natural history of genital herpes is a primary infection followed by episodes of recurrence. The virus lies dormant in the dorsal root ganglia of the spinal cord and reactivation causes recurrent symptoms. There are two distinct types of the virus: HSV-1 (typically causing cold sores around the mouth) and HSV-2 (almost exclusively associated with infection in the genital area). In the UK, these types probably contribute equally to the prevalence of genital herpes,[7] although HSV-2 generally causes more severe and frequently recurrent symptoms.

Transmission is through direct contact and risk is greatest during a symptomatic episode, but asymptomatic viral shedding also occurs, occurring in 80% of people with HSV-2.[7] Once transmission has occurred, primary infection usually develops 4–7 days later, with painful genital ulceration, dysuria, vaginal or urethral discharge and sometimes urinary retention. The primary infection is usually the most severe and the patient may also feel systemically unwell. Classical signs include erythema, blistering and ulceration of the genitals and surrounding areas, and inguinal lymph nodes may be enlarged and tender.

If a diagnosis of HSV is suspected, urgent referral to the local genitourinary service would be appropriate for further investigation and treatment. Viral culture should ideally be carried out on all patients with a first episode of genital herpes and is highly sensitive and specific. Swabs are taken from blistered lesions to collect any vesicle fluid, and virus-infected cells are scraped from the base of the blister.

There is no cure for genital herpes, although it is usually self-limiting. Primary episodes should be treated with oral antiviral medication for a minimum of five days, or until no new lesions are forming. Treatment of recurrent episodes is dependent upon symptoms and severity.

Trichomoniasis is caused by a flagellated protozoan, *Trichomonas vaginalis*, and involves the vagina, urethra and para-urethral glands. Typical symptoms include vaginal discharge, vulval itching, dysuria and offensive odour, although symptoms may be absent in 50% of women.[8] Signs are present in 85%–95% of women with trichomoniasis and include a vaginal discharge (which may be thin and scanty, or thick, profuse, frothy and yellow-green), inflammation of the vagina and vulva and a strawberry appearance of the cervix in 2% of cases.

Genitourinary service referral, with microscopic examination of a wet smear from a high vaginal swab, can diagnose 40%–80% of infected women.[8] Diagnosis by culture increases detection rate to 95% but is not usually routinely available. The treatment of choice is oral metronidazole.

PID is a clinical diagnosis and results from spread of infection from the lower to the upper genital tract, involving the uterus, fallopian tubes and ovaries. The main causative organisms are *Chlamydia trachomatis*, less commonly *Neisseria gonorrhoeae* and *Mycoplasma genitalium*, and *Gardnerella vaginalis*; Gram-negative organisms can also be involved.[9]

No single symptom or sign is specifically diagnostic of PID. Typical symptoms include lower abdominal pain, dyspareunia, abnormal vaginal bleeding, abnormal vaginal discharge and dysuria.[10] On examination, cervical motion tenderness and adnexal tenderness are typical; a mucopurulent cervical discharge and cervicitis may be seen on speculum examination and the patient may be pyrexial.

Cervical swabs for *Chlamydia trachomatis* and *Neisseria gonorrhoeae* are recommended, although negative swabs do not exclude a diagnosis of PID and treatment should always be commenced if there are clinical signs. Delay in treatment could lead to complications such as tubal infertility (affecting around 10% of women with a history of PID), ectopic pregnancy (1–5%) and chronic pelvic pain (30%).[10]

Antibiotic treatment should cover *Chlamydia trachomatis*, *Neisseria gonorrhoeae* and anaerobes for 14 days. If after this time symptoms and signs are still present, a further 14 days of treatment is usually administered.

Others

Genital warts are common; they are caused by a small DNA virus – a papillomavirus – most commonly human papillomavirus, of which more than 80 types exist. Thirty types are associated with genital infection, usually type 6 or 11. Transmission is by skin-to-skin contact and the incubation period is from two weeks to eight months, sometimes longer.

Diagnosis is clinical and treatment of external warts is purely cosmetic, initially with locally applied caustic agents such as podophyllin.

Syphilis is caused by a spirochaete, *Treponema pallidum*, and is classified as primary or secondary. Primary syphilis typically presents as an ulcer (or chancre) and regional lymphadenopathy 9–90 days after exposure. Secondary syphilis presents with multisystem disease within the first two years of infection. Diagnosis is serological and treatment is with long-acting penicillin.

Details of HIV and hepatitis infections are not described here but need consideration as part of a full sexual health screen.

Recent Developments

Sexually transmitted diseases are a public health issue. Thus, on diagnosis or suspicion of an STI, referral to the local genitourinary service for more comprehensive screening and follow-up is advisable. Patients should always be advised to avoid sexual intercourse during treatment and current partners also need to be treated. Contact tracing is essential to control spread of infection throughout the community, and follow-up to ensure compliance and resolution of symptoms may also be appropriate.

Conclusion

Provision of combined sexual health and contraceptive services are essential for this patient. She also needs to be advised to use effective contraception to avoid an unplanned pregnancy.

Further Reading

1 Centers for Disease Control and Prevention. Trends in Reportable Sexually Transmitted Diseases in the United States, 2005. www.cdc.gov/std/stats/trends2005.htm (accessed 17 09 07)

2 Health Protection Agency. *Diagnoses of selected STIs by region, sex and age group, United Kingdom: 1996–2005.* HPA, 2006.

3 Department of Health. *The national strategy for sexual health and HIV.* London: Department of Health, 2001. www.dh.gov.uk/en/Publicationsandstatistics/Publications/PublicationsPolicyAndGuidance/DH_4003133 (accessed 17 09 07)

4 Kinghorn G. A sexual health and HIV strategy for England. *BMJ* 2001; **323**: 243–4.

5 CKS Clinical topic. Chlamydia – uncomplicated, genital (women). www.cks.library.nhs.uk/chlamydia_uncomplicated_genital (accessed 17 09 07)

6 Clinical Effectiveness Group (Association for Genitourinary Medicine and the Medical Society for the Study of Venereal Diseases). National guideline on the diagnosis and treatment of gonorrhoea in adults (2005). www.bashh.org/guidelines/2005/gc_final_0805.pdf (accessed 17 09 07)

7 CKS Clinical topic. Herpes simplex – genital.
www.cks.library.nhs.uk/herpes_simplex_genital (accessed 17 09 07)

8 CKS Clinical topic. Trichomonas. www.cks.library.nhs.uk/trichomoniasis (accessed 17 09 07)

9 Clinical Effectiveness Group (Association for Genitourinary Medicine and the Medical Society for the Study of Venereal Diseases). National guideline for the management of pelvic inflammatory disease (2005). www.bashh.org/guidelines/2005/pid_v4_0205.pdf (accessed 17 09 07)

10 CKS Clinical topic. Pelvic inflammatory disease.
www.cks.library.nhs.uk/pelvic_inflammatory_disease (accessed 17 09 07)

PROBLEM

36 Stress Incontinence

Case History

A 33-year-old solicitor complains of highly embarrassing urinary incontinence. She has had two children in the past five years and has noticed slight leakage of urine when exercising, coughing or sneezing since midterm in her first pregnancy. Recently she has felt a dragging sensation when walking, and has had one episode of serious incontinence at work.

What are relevant questions and what should you examine for?

What are the conservative options?

What are the surgical options?

Background

It has been estimated that 20%–30% of the female population experience involuntary leakage of urine. Urodynamic stress incontinence is defined as the involuntary loss of urine when the intravesical pressure exceeds the maximum urethral closure pressure in the absence of detrusor overactivity. The bladder neck and proximal urethra are intra-abdominal organs, supported by the pubo-urethral ligaments. If the ligaments are damaged, or the pelvic floor sags, the proximal urethra slips through and leakage of urine can occur. Risk factors for stress urinary incontinence are shown in Table 36.1.

Table 36.1 Risk factors for stress urinary incontinence

- Female sex: women 2–3 times more common than men

- Age: incontinence can occur at any age but is much more common at >70 years

- Pregnancy and childbirth: pregnancy puts an enormous strain on the pelvic floor, as does a vaginal birth, large baby, prolonged second stage and forceps. A Caesarean section does not prevent incontinence

- Menopause: the drop in oestrogens affects the collagen of the pelvic floor making the fascia and ligaments weaker; this leads to prolapse and incontinence

- Smoking: increases the risk 2- to 3-fold; women who smoke have an earlier menopause by 2–3 years and also raise their intra-abdominal pressures by coughing

- Obesity: because of raised intra-abdominal pressure

What are relevant questions and what should you examine for?

History and examination should focus on the following.
Questions to ask her:

- Is there any pain/blood when passing urine?

- How often do you pass urine a day?

- How often do you pass urine at night?

- Do you wear a pad? How often do you change it?

The examination should:

- Exclude a urinary tract infection/diabetes by testing urine

- Exclude an abdominal or pelvic mass: investigate appropriately

- Exclude a full bladder (urinary outflow obstruction)

- Check for prolapse by asking the woman to bear down whilst examining her

- Look at the tissues for atrophic vaginitis

- Assess pelvic floor strength by asking the woman to grip on gloved finger in vagina

- Include a full neurological examination if appropriate

What are the conservative options?

Conservative measures are used as first-line options, as they may help and do no harm. They are also useful for women who do not want a surgical option, either because they do not have the time to have a surgical procedure, or have not finished their families, are unfit or are already on a waiting list.

Pelvic floor muscle training

From a meta-analysis of 43 trials,[1] pelvic floor muscle training (PFMT) was better than no treatment or placebo treatments for women with stress or mixed incontinence. 'Intensive' PFMT appeared to be better than 'standard' PFMT. PFMT may be more effective than some types of electrical stimulation but there were problems in combining the data from these trials. There is insufficient evidence to determine if PFMT is better or worse than other treatments, as there are very few head-to-head trials. The effect of adding PFMT to other treatments (e.g. electrical stimulation, behavioural training) is not clear due to the limited amount of evidence available. Evidence of the effect of adding other adjunctive treatments to PFMT (e.g. vaginal cones, intravaginal resistance) is equally limited. The effectiveness of biofeedback-assisted PFMT is not clear, but on the basis of the evidence available there did not appear to be any benefit over PFMT alone at post-treatment assessment. Long-term outcomes of PFMT are unclear. Side effects of PFMT were uncommon and reversible.

Given that we know pregnancy and childbirth are the major risk factor for stress incontinence, should we focus our attention to preventative measures and teach and encourage all women to do pelvic floor exercises during pregnancy? In a study of twelve trials, antepartum PFMT, when used with biofeedback and taught by trained healthcare personnel, using a conservative model, does not result in a significant short-term (three months) decrease in post-partum urinary incontinence or pelvic floor strength.[2] Post-partum PFMT, when performed with a vaginal device providing resistance or feedback, appears to decrease post-partum urinary incontinence and to increase pelvic floor strength.[2] There are difficulties with all the reported trials of small numbers and heterogeneity of methods used.

Local oestrogens

In post-menopausal women with atrophic vaginitis, local oestrogen replacement with oestrogen cream, pessaries or a ring can be an option. These local oestradiol preparations do not carry the risks of increased breast cancer as they are not systemically absorbed. Any post-menopausal bleeding should be investigated, as in any woman with a uterus.

Taking all trials in a meta-analysis,[3] the data suggested that about 50% of women treated with oestrogen were cured or improved compared with about 25% on placebo. The effect was actually larger for urge incontinence than for stress incontinence.

Duloxetine

Duloxetine is a combined serotonin and noradrenaline reuptake inhibitor (SNRI) that improves continence in women with stress incontinence, probably by increasing muscle tone in the urethra during bladder filling.[4] It interacts with antidepressants such as monoamine oxidase inhibitors and fluvoxamine as well as drugs that increase the risk of bleeding. Special precautions should be taken if there is a past medical history of seizures, manic depression or suicidal ideation, or glaucoma or raised intra-ocular pressure. It can cause insomnia, nausea, thirst, headache, blurred vision and muscle weakness.

Urodynamic studies

It is often difficult to know what is going on in a woman with urinary incontinence, and sometimes there is a mixed picture. If simple exercises fail, a referral for full urodynamic studies should be made to a specialist urogynaecology centre to take the patient to an accurate diagnosis.

What are the surgical options?

Surgery (Table 36.2) always carries the risks of infection, death from anaesthesia or the sequelae of post-operative immobility. Also there is a woeful lack of data on long-term

Table 36.2 Surgical procedures for stress incontinence
Anterior colporrhaphy   Poor success rate
Marshall-Marchetti-Krantz   Does not treat cystocoele
Burch colposuspension   Good ten-year data; corrects stress incontinence and cystocoele; can do hysterectomy at same time
Tension-free vaginal tapes   Can do under spinal anaesthesia as day case; long-term data lacking
Injectables (macroplastiques, glutaraldehyde cross-linked [GAX] collagen, collagen GAX, collagen)   Done cystoscopically; 50% two-year cure-rate data

(over five years) outcomes on any of the newer surgical sling procedures for stress incontinence.

Thirteen trials were identified including 760 women of whom 627 were treated with suburethral slings.[5] Five trials compared suburethral slings with open abdominal retropubic colposuspension (Burch/Marshall-Marchetti-Krantz) and one compared suburethral slings with needle suspension (Stamey). In six trials, different types of suburethral sling were compared with each other. Nine types of slings were included: Teflon, polytetrafluoroethylene, prolene used for transvaginal tape, porcine dermis, lyophilized dura mater, fascia lata, vaginal wall, autologous dermis and rectus fascia. There were no comparisons of suburethral sling with anterior repair, laparoscopic retropubic suspension, peri-urethral injections or artificial sphincters. One trial compared surgery (including slings) with anticholinergic medication. There were no statistically significant differences between traditional slings and other types of continence surgery, or between one type of traditional sling and another sling. Confidence intervals around the estimates were wide, reflecting the few data available, and so clinically important differences could not be ruled out. Reliable evidence on which to judge whether or not suburethral slings are better or worse than other surgical or conservative management is currently not available.[5] From tension-free vaginal tape (TVT) sling operations, the continence rate in a series of 99 women was 80% at one year.[6] Cystotomy can occur in 14.4% of TVT procedures, but rather comfortingly does not appear to adversely affect clinical outcome.[7] There are long-term follow-up (10–14 years) data on Burch colposuspension: 55.3% of women were still dry a decade later in Taiwan,[8] but only 19% in Sweden after 14 years.[9] Both groups still had considerable lower urinary tract irritability. Patients must be counselled prior to surgery that they understand the procedure might make them worse or no better, and may not be the long-term solution they were hoping for.

Recent Developments

Periurethral or transurethral injection of bulking agents is another surgical procedure for the treatment of stress urinary incontinence. A systematic review found that silicone particles, calcium hydroxylapatite, ethylene vinyl alcohol and carbon spheres gave improvements equivalent to collagen. Porcine dermal implant gave improvements comparable to silicone at six months.[10] A comparison of periurethral and transurethral methods of delivery of the bulking agent found a similar outcome but a higher rate of early complications in the periurethral group. The authors concluded that injection therapy may represent a useful option for short-term symptomatic relief amongst selected women with co-morbidity that precludes anaesthesia – two or three injections are likely to be required to achieve a satisfactory result.

Conclusion

The option that this patient will opt for will depend on her desire for further children. It is likely that she will start by using pelvic floor exercises or drug treatment.

Further Reading

1 Hay-Smith EJ, Bo K, Berghmans LC, Hendriks HJ, de Bie RA, van Waalwijk van Doorn ES. Pelvic floor muscle training for urinary incontinence in women. *Cochrane Database Syst Rev* 2001; CD001407.

2 Harvey MA. Pelvic floor exercises during and after pregnancy: a systematic review of their role in preventing pelvic floor dysfunction. *J Obstet Gynaecol Can* 2003; **25**: 487–98.

3 Moehrer B, Hextall A, Jackson S. Oestrogens for urinary incontinence in women. *Cochrane Database Syst Rev* 2003; CD001405.

4 Mariappan P, Alhasso A, Ballantyne Z, Grant A, N'Dow J. Duloxetine, a serotonin and noradrenaline reuptake inhibitor (SNRI) for the treatment of stress urinary incontinence: a systematic review. *Eur Urol* 2007; **51**: 67–74.

5 Bezerra CA, Bruschini H, Cody DJ. Traditional suburethral sling operations for urinary incontinence in women. *Cochrane Database Syst Rev* 2005; CD001754.

6 Bjelic-Radisic V, Dorfer M, Greimel E, Frudinger A, Tamussino K, Winter R. Quality of life and continence 1 year after the tension-free vaginal tape operation. *Am J Obstet Gynecol* 2006; **195**: 1784–8.

7 LaSala CA, Schimpf MO, Udoh E, O'Sullivan DM, Tulikangas P. Outcome of tension-free vaginal tape procedure when complicated by intraoperative cystotomy. *Am J Obstet Gynecol* 2006; **195**: 1857–61.

8 Ng S, Tee YT, Tsui KP, Chen GD. Is the role of Burch colposuspension fading away in this epoch for treating female urinary incontinence? *Int Urogynecol J Pelvic Floor Dysfunct* 2006; [Epub ahead of print].

9 Kjolhede P. Long-term efficacy of Burch colposuspension: a 14-year follow-up study. *Acta Obstet Gynecol Scand* 2005; **84**: 767–72.

10 Keegan P, Atiemo K, Cody J, McClinton S, Pickard R. Periurethral injection therapy for urinary incontinence in women. *Cochrane Database Syst Rev* 2007; CD003881.

37 Urge Incontinence

Case History

A 68-year-old retired social worker has found that recently she has been incontinent of urine. It has happened when out shopping and she felt she wanted to go, but was unable to control her bladder long enough to find a public toilet in time. This has since got worse and she is passing urine in her pants 3–4 times a day. She is mortified, and wants to stay with her married daughter over Christmas, but is too ashamed to accept the invitation in case she wets the bed.

What are relevant questions and what should you examine for?

What are the drug options?

How are the drug options tolerated?

Background

About 50–100 million people are estimated to be affected by an overactive bladder (OAB),[1] which has a prevalence of about 16% in people aged over 40 years.[2] OAB is a chronic condition defined urodynamically as detrusor overactivity, and characterized by involuntary bladder contractions during the filling phase of the micturition cycle.[3] However, clinically in primary care without access to a urodynamic laboratory, a few key questions can define the constellation of symptoms, as long as other factors such as metabolic abnormalities (e.g. diabetes, hypercalcaemia) or urinary pathology (e.g. urinary tract infections, interstitial cystitis, stones) have been excluded.

From a study of 16 776 subjects in six different European countries, the prevalence of OAB symptoms was 16.6% in people (men and women) of age 40 years and over.[2] The prevalence increased with age: in men, increasing slowly to age 69 years, then increasing sharply after 75 years; in women, increasing slowly to age 59 years, then levelling in the 60s and increasing sharply at age 70 and above. Of those that reported symptoms, 85% had urinary frequency, 54% urgency and 36% urge incontinence. Rather surprisingly, 60% had consulted a doctor about their symptoms, but only 27% were currently being treated. The commonest reason for not consulting was the belief that no help was available.

An OAB has a severe impact on quality of life.[4] Sleep disturbance may result in daytime somnolence, reduced cognitive function, and impaired concentration causing errors at work and driving. The relentless restrictions on lifestyle cause high depression scores and low self-esteem. Untreated OAB is associated with an increased risk of urinary tract infections, skin infections from constant wet and chafing pads, and injury from falls in the elderly when people attempt to rush to the toilet and trip. In all, 65% of OAB patients said that their symptoms adversely affected their daily lives.[2]

What are relevant questions and what should you examine for?

It takes a lot of courage for people to seek help. Although an OAB profoundly affects quality of life,[4] people do not even discuss these issues with their partner. Patients need to feel confident they are taken seriously, and listened to. It may take more than one consultation to undertake the full history and examination (Tables 37.1 and 37.2), as often such discussions are blurted out at the end of a consultation about something else. There may be a mixture of stress and urge incontinence symptoms that are difficult to clarify, and patients may not be completely honest about their symptoms as they are too ashamed even to admit these to a sympathetic nurse or doctor. You need to ask:

Table 37.1 The key clinical history features to distinguish the different types of incontinence	
Frequency	Urinate >8 times a day Urinate >2 times at night
Urgency	Have a strong urge to pass urine with no advance warning Have to run to get to toilet in time Have to keep running to the toilet
Urge incontinence	Unable to get to toilet in time Sudden and uncontrolled loss of urine Urinary leakage during day Urinary leakage at night when asleep
Stress incontinence	Leakage when sneezing or laughing Leakage exercising or bending Leakage lifting or pulling
Outflow obstruction	Even when wanting to urinate, trouble getting started Weak stream when urinating Dribbling after stopping urinating

Source: modified from Milsom et al. 2001.[2]

Table 37.2 Examination
• Exclude an abdominal or pelvic mass (including pregnancy)
• Exclude a full bladder (obstruction/retention)
• Check for prolapse
• Check for post-menopausal atrophy
• Pelvic floor strength
• Neurological examination if indicated[*]
• Exclude a urinary tract infection/haematuria with a urinalysis dipstick and send for MSU if appropriate

* If the story sounds like denervation due to a slipped disc, trauma or some progressive neurological disease (e.g. multiple sclerosis), then an appropriate neurological examination should be performed and/or a neurological opinion sought.

- Is there pain/blood passing urine?

- How often are you passing urine in a day?

- How often are you passing urine at night?

- Do you get any warning before the incontinence?

What are the drug options?

Anticholinergic drugs – darifenacin, oxybutynin, propiverine, tolterodine, trospium chloride and solifenacin – block the parasympathetic nerves which control bladder emptying and have a direct relaxing effect on the detrusor muscle. They all lower intravesicular pressure, increase capacity and reduce the frequency of bladder contractions, so helping to reduce incontinence. They are all contraindicated in patients with glaucoma or at risk of glaucoma. Many patients do not like the side effects of these drugs such as nausea, blurred vision, a very dry mouth and constipation. Palpitations are also frequent. Patients must be warned of these side effects, and often by starting at a very low dose and working up over about a month, people can adjust to the drug.
Doses (in adults):

- Darifenacin   7.5–15 mg once daily

- Oxybutynin   5 mg twice or four times daily

- Propiverine   15 mg twice or four times daily

- Tolterodine   2 mg twice daily

- Trospium chloride   20 mg twice daily

- Solifenacin   5 mg once daily

It is often difficult to know what is going on in a woman with urinary incontinence, and sometimes there is a mixed picture. If simple exercises teaching the patient to resist and inhibit the sensation of urgency and a trial of medication fail, a referral for full urodynamic studies should be made to a specialist urogynaecology centre to take the patient to an accurate diagnosis.

How are the drug options tolerated?

In two studies in which patients were treated with tolterodine 2 mg twice daily for 9–12 months, the completion rates were 70% and 62%, respectively, with adverse events in 9% and 15% of patients.[5-7] In a study using extended-release oxybutynin for twelve months,[8] 54% of patients stopped treatment, 24% because of adverse events. In a year-long study of trospium chloride, again about 25% of patients stopped the study, 6% due to adverse advents.[9] In a 52-week study (40-week open-label extension of a two 12-week, placebo-controlled, double-blind trial) with solifenacin at 5 mg or 10 mg daily, there was a 19% dropout rate, with 4.7% of patients discontinuing for adverse events,[10] the same as placebo.[5] Efficacy of solifenacin was observed within one week of treatment, but stabilized over twelve weeks. After twelve weeks' treatment, 50% of those who had experienced incontinence before treatment were free of incontinent episodes, and 35% achieved a micturition frequency of less than eight voids per day. Treatment also resulted in improvement in quality of life measures: general health perception, incontinence impact, role limitations, physical limitations, social limitations, emotions, symptom severity and sleep/energy levels.[10]

Recent Developments

Botulinum toxin (BTX) can be injected directly into the muscle and inhibits acetyl-choline at the presynaptic junction. This paralyses the muscle in the short term and leads to long-term atrophy. A study of 15 patients with OAB who had not responded to anti-cholinergics showed BTX injections produced a 76% resolution of urgency within two weeks which lasted an average of nine months.[11] Other studies have shown similar results.[12] Long-term studies on cost-effectiveness, safety and efficacy are required.

Conclusion

This woman's investigations have proved to be normal and she has elected to try drug therapy as this is not contraindicated by concomitant disease or medication. If a trial of medication fails she will need to be referred for urodynamic studies.

Further Reading

1 Kelleher CJ, Cardozo L, Chapple CR, Haab F, Ridder AM. Improved quality of life in patients with overactive bladder symptoms treated with solifenacin. *BJU Int* 2005; **95**: 81–5.

2 Milsom I, Abrams P, Cardozo L, Roberts R, Thuroff J, Wein A. How widespread are the symptoms of an overactive bladder and how are they managed? A population-based prevalence study. *BJU Int* 2001; **87**: 760–6.

3 Abrams P, Blaivas J, Stanton S, Andersen J. The standardisation of terminology of lower urinary tract function. *Neurourol Urodyn* 1988; **7**: 403–27.

4 Jackson S. The patient with an overactive bladder – symptoms and quality-of-life issues. *Urology* 1997; **50** (6A Suppl): 18–22.

5 Chapple CR, Rechberger T, Al-Shukri S, Meffan P, Everaert K, Huang M, Ridder A: YM-905 Study Group. Randomized, double-blind placebo- and tolterodine-controlled trial of the once-daily antimuscarinic agent solifenacin in patients with symptomatic overactive bladder. *BJU Int* 2004; **93**: 303–10.

6 Abrams P, Malone-Lee J, Jacquetin B, Wyndaele JJ, Tammela T, Jonas U, Wein A. Twelve-month treatment of overactive bladder: efficacy and tolerability of tolterodine. *Drugs Aging* 2001; **18**: 551–60.

7 Appell RA, Abrams P, Drutz HP, Van Kerrebroeck PE, Millard R, Wein A. Treatment of overactive bladder: long-term tolerability and efficacy of tolterodine. *World J Urol* 2001; **19**: 141–7.

8 Diokno A, Sand P, Labasky R, Sieber P, Antoci J, Leach G, Atkinson L, Albrecht D. Long-term safety of extended-release oxybutynin chloride in a community-dwelling population of participants with overactive bladder: a one-year study. *Int Urol Nephrol* 2002; **34**: 43–9.

9 Halaska M, Ralph G, Wiedemann A, Primus G, Ballering-Brühl B, Höfner K, Jonas U. Controlled, double-blind, multicentre clinical trial to investigate long-term tolerability and efficacy of trospium chloride in patients with detrusor instability. *World J Urol* 2003: **20**: 392–9.

10 Haab F, Cardozo L, Chapple C, Ridder AM: Solifenacin Study Group. Long-term open-label solifenacin treatment associated with persistence with therapy in patients with overactive bladder syndrome. *Eur Urol* 2005; **47**: 376–84.

11 Rajkumar GN, Small DR, Mustafa AW, Conn G. A prospective study to evaluate safety, tolerability, efficacy and durability of response of intravesical injection of botulinum toxin type A into detrusor muscle in patients with refractory idiopathic detrusor overactivity. *BJU Int* 2005; **96**: 848–52.

12 Sahai A, Khan MS, Dasgupta P. Efficacy of botulinum toxin-A for treating idiopathic detrusor overactivity: results from a single center, randomized, double-blind, placebo controlled trial. *J Urol* 2007; **177**: 2231–6.

PROBLEM

38 Recurrent Urinary Tract Infections

Case History

Miss P, aged 36 years, attends on Monday morning with haematuria, frequency and dysuria. She has been up all night with these symptoms and feels too ill to teach her classes. She has no loin pain and is mid-cycle. She uses condoms and a spermicide for contraception and has spent the weekend visiting her boyfriend in London. She is annoyed as this is the fourth time she has had this trouble in the past year. She is otherwise well but smokes 20 cigarettes a day.

What should you ask and what tests should you do?

What causes recurrent urinary tract infections (UTIs)?

What are the treatment options?

What are special considerations?

What are long-term management strategies?

Background

Cystitis is an inflammation of the lining of the bladder. It can be caused by a variety of inflammatory agents, such as a bacterial infection. Some women have significant bacteriuria without symptoms; this is known as asymptomatic bacteriuria. An uncomplicated urinary tract infection (UTI) is an infection in the bladder only in an otherwise well woman with no abnormality of her urinary tract and no predisposing factors (see Table 38.1). A complicated UTI is in a patient with anatomical or metabolic factors. All infections of the kidney (upper urinary tract) are regarded as complicated, as are those of men or children. A distinction also needs to be made between relapse (persistence of same pathogen in the urinary tract) or reinfection (the acquisition of a new pathogen). Kass, in the 1950s, quantitatively assessed the number of colony-forming bacteria per millilitre of voided urine in acute pyelonephritis in children. From his work, 10^5 colony-forming units (CFU) has now been adopted in laboratories around the world as an arbitrary cut-off, although Stamm has argued that this has a low sensitivity for ordinary UTIs and that 10^2 CFU is a more sensitive indicator of symptomatic UTIs in women.[1] Certainly a lot of symptomatic women are told their urine culture is 'normal' in primary care, when what is actually meant is that they have less than 10^5 CFU; clinically this can cause confusion.

Table 38.1 Risk factors for upper urinary tract infection
Physiological Pregnancy Diabetes mellitus Urogenital ageing
Anatomical Urinary tract abnormality: congenital or acquired Urinary stone Surgical instrumentation Indwelling foreign body (stent or catheter)
Past medical history Recurrent UTIs Previous pyelonephritis Immunosuppression

What should you ask and what tests should you do?

The key questions are:

- How often are you passing water during the day, and at night?

- Does it hurt? (Where?)

- How soon did these symptoms start after sexual intercourse?

- How long have you and your partner been together?

Dipstick testing. Testing a mid-stream urine sample with a leukocyte esterase and nitrite dipstick has a sensitivity of 75%–99% predicting culture-proven infection.[1] Antibiotics should be prescribed to those with a positive test. Mid-stream urine (MSU) samples should be sent for analysis in all recurrent or complicated UTIs, and therapy adjusted in the light of clinical response and laboratory information on sensitivities.

MSU samples. Medical practice so often flounders when simple basics are not discussed with patients. An MSU sample is required. These are often contaminated with mixed faecal and skin flora, which renders the information useless, as the urine dribbles over the perineum to get in the pot. It has been shown in ambulatory patients that extensive perineal cleansing and a sterile pot are not prerequisites for a decent MSU sample, but simply parting the labia with one hand whilst holding the pot in the other to get a clean-catch midstream urine sample significantly reduces contamination. Ideally, the specimen should then be plated-up in the laboratory within two hours, rather than incubating on an office shelf for another eight hours before reaching the laboratory. Such things make a difference.

Further imaging. In women with recurrent UTIs (more than two in 6 months or three in 12 months), an underlying obstructive uropathy, congenital abnormality or stone must be excluded. However, on ultrasound scan, intravenous pyelography or cystoscopy, fewer than 5% of patients have a demonstrable abnormality.[1]

What causes recurrent UTIs?

Bacteria gain access to the bladder from ascending the short female urethra. Lymphatic or haematogenous spread is exceedingly rare. Infection is determined by the size of the inoculum, host resistance and defence systems, and the virulence of the pathogen. Urine inhibits bacterial growth due to its osmolarity, high urea content and low pH, and frequent flushing of the bladder by urination can wash bacteria out. Tamm–Horsfall proteins competitively inhibit *Escherichia coli* attachment to the surface of the bladder. The vaginal commensal lactobacilli interfere with *E.coli* adhesions, so protecting from infection, as does the mucopolysaccharide coating of the transitional epithelial cells of the bladder mucosa.

What are the treatment options?

Fluid intake. Many women in busy offices, especially if they have a distaste for using shared toilets, do not drink enough fluid. This may predispose to urinary stones and UTIs. Conversely, some have argued that the 'drink as much as you can' approach when women have a UTI may make things worse by enhancing vesicoureteral reflux and diluting the antibacterial substances in the urine when they are prescribed. There is no prospective trial on this.

Self-help. Cranberry juice has been shown to inhibit pathogenic *E.coli* fimbriae, with a high molecular weight inhibitor of adhesin. Small (30 ml) doses of cranberry juice taken before bed have been shown to reduce the number of recurrent UTIs in elderly women in residential care settings.

Antibiotics (Table 38.2). Consideration must always be given to specific allergies and if the woman may be pregnant or breast-feeding. Broad-spectrum antibiotics may reduce the efficacy of oral contraception and the woman must be advised to use condoms too if appropriate.

What are special considerations?

Pregnancy. The patient must be asked whether she is pregnant or might be pregnant. Pregnant women have a higher rate of asymptomatic bacteriuria. Obstetric complications of UTIs include premature labour, small-for-dates babies and increased perinatal mortality. Asymptomatic bacteriuria also needs treating.

Table 38.2 Antibiotics used in urinary tract infections

Antibiotic	Advantages	Disadvantages
Trimethoprim	Cheap; effective in 78% CAIs	22% CAIs resistant; folate antagonist in pregnancy (avoid in first trimester)
Cephalosporins	Effective in 87.5% CAIs	More expensive; more side effects (thrush etc.)
Ampicillin/Amoxicillin	Safe in pregnancy and breast-feeding	40% CAIs resistant
Co-amoxiclav	Effective in 87.5% CAIs	Manufacturers advise avoid in pregnancy unless essential, but no evidence of teratogenicity
Nitrofurantoin	Cheap; effective in 88.4% CAIs; can be used in pregnancy, but may cause neonatal haemolysis at birth	Side effect of nausea and vomiting
Quinolones	91.5% effective in UK (some countries where OTC, now <60% sensitive)	Expensive; cannot be used in pregnancy; caution with epilepsy or hepatic/renal impairment

CAIs, community acquired infections; UK, United Kingdom; OTC, over the counter.

Diabetes mellitus. Asymptomatic bacteriuria is 40 times more common in diabetic than in non-diabetic women. High urinary glucose impairs leukocyte phagocytosis. Up to 50% of cases may have upper urinary tract involvement.

Stones. A stone acts as a focus for bacterial persistence. *Proteus mirabilis* is a more common pathogen. It is impossible to 'cure' a UTI in the presence of a stone, and urological treatment by ultrasonic disruption or surgical removal of the calculus must be considered.

Urogenital ageing. Local oestrogen cream or pessaries significantly reduce the recurrence of UTIs if urogenital ageing is a problem.

What are long-term management strategies?

In non-pregnant women with recurrent UTIs, continuous low-dose antibiotic prophylaxis (i.e. nitrofurantoin 50 mg at night) for 6–12 months reduced the rate of UTI when compared to placebo, although there were more adverse events in the antibiotic group, and UTI rates returned to previous levels after the 6 months of low-dose antibiotics were stopped.[2] One randomized controlled trial compared post-coital versus continuous daily ciprofloxacin and found no significant difference in rates of UTIs, suggesting that a three-day post-coital treatment could be offered to women who have UTI associated with sexual intercourse. The usage of spermicide-containing products and/or a poorly fitted diaphragm may also contribute to a post-coital infection.[3] Patients can effectively diagnose their own UTIs and self-initiate treatments with the same success rate as their doctors. Allowing women to have several courses of antibiotics to take 'as and when required' is a reasonable option, as long as they are reviewed at six months (Figure 38.1).

In pregnant women, antibiotic treatment is effective for the cure of UTIs, but there are insufficient data to recommend any specific treatment regimen for symptomatic UTIs during pregnancy.[4] Randomized trials comparing antibiotic treatment with placebo or no treatment in pregnant women with asymptomatic bacteriuria found on antenatal screening, showed that antibiotic treatment reduced the incidence of pyelonephritis, preterm delivery and low birth weight babies.[5]

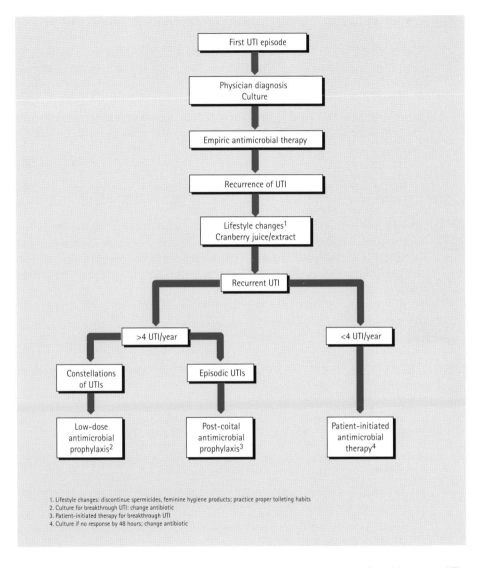

Figure 38.1 A proposed treatment algorithm for pre-menopausal women presenting with recurrent UTI. *Source*: Nickel 2005 (with permission).[9]

Recent Developments

The increasing microbial antibiotic resistance motivates research for non-antibiotic treatment alternatives. In recurrent UTIs, 'bacterial interference' has attracted interest as a possible alternative treatment option. The observation that asymptomatic bacteriuria protects against recurrent UTI has prompted clinical trials with deliberate colonization of the human urinary tract as an alternative approach in patients with recurrent UTI.[6,7] Many *in vitro* studies, animal experiments, microbiological studies in healthy women and clinical trials in women with UTIs have been carried out to assess the effectiveness and safety of probiotics for prophylaxis against uropathogens. Most of the studies had encouraging findings for some specific strains of lactobacilli.[8] The evidence from the available studies suggests that probiotics can be beneficial for preventing recurrent UTIs in women; they also have a good safety profile. However, further research is needed to confirm these results before the widespread use of probiotics for this indication can be recommended.

Conclusion

This patient has had four episodes over the past year. She needs an MSU sent for analysis. One should consider imaging. Her episodes are post-coital and she uses a spermicide for contraception. She should consider post-coital antibiotic prophylaxis and changing her form of contraception, for example, to a progesterone-only pill since she is over 35 years old and smokes.

Further Reading

1 Stamm WE, Hooton TM. Management of urinary tract infections in adults. *N Engl J Med* 1993; **329**: 1328–34.

2 Albert X, Huertas I, Pereiró I, Sanfélix J, Gosalbes V, Perrota C. Antibiotics for preventing recurrent urinary tract infection in non-pregnant women. *Cochrane Database Syst Rev* 2004; CD001209.

3 Hooton TM. Recurrent urinary tract infection in women. *Int J Antimicrob Agents* 2001; **17**: 259–68.

4 Vazquez JC, Villar J. Treatments for symptomatic urinary tract infections during pregnancy. *Cochrane Database Syst Rev* 2003; CD002256.

5 Smaill F. Antibiotics for asymptomatic bacteriuria in pregnancy. *Cochrane Database Syst Rev* 2001; CD000490.

6 Darouiche RO, Hull RA. Bacterial interference for prevention of urinary tract infection: an overview. *J Spinal Cord Med* 2000; **23**: 136–41.

7 Sundén F, Håkansson L, Ljunggren E, Wullt B. Bacterial interference – is deliberate colonization with *Escherichia coli* 83972 an alternative treatment for patients with recurrent urinary tract infection? *Int J Antimicrob Agents* 2006; **28** (Suppl 1): S26–9.

8 Falagas ME, Betsi GI, Tokas T, Athanasiou S. Probiotics for prevention of recurrent urinary tract infections in women: a review of the evidence from microbiological and clinical studies. *Drugs* 2006; **66**: 1253–61.

9 Nickel JC. Practical management of recurrent urinary tract infections in premenopausal women. *Rev Urol* 2005; **7**: 11–17.

39 Chronic Interstitial Cystitis

Case History

A 34-year-old woman comes into your consulting room. She says she is fed up with the entire medical profession as her life has been ruined by urinary frequency and urgency. She cannot go out, unless she knows where all the public conveniences are, and makes excuses to the few friends she still has when they invite her somewhere. She has broken up with her boyfriend as sex seemed painful and made her symptoms worse. She has not had a decent night's sleep for three years because of nocturia. She has consulted countless other doctors who 'cannot find anything wrong' and suggested she seeks psychiatric help. She admits she is now suicidal, but only because she feels she has no quality of life and no prospects of getting better (at this point of the consultation she is crying so hard she can no longer talk).

What are relevant questions?

What are relevant tests?

What treatments are available?

Background

Chronic interstitial cystitis (IC) is one of those tricky fields of medicine where there is no consensus of symptoms to make a diagnosis, no easy standard test to confirm that diagnosis and, as the aetiology is unknown, all the treatments are empirical and have varying success rates from 'modest' to 'poor'. It is not surprising that the group of people that end up with this diagnosis are disgruntled, if not suicidal. There are also areas of overlap with other diseases that cause pelvic pain, and some women may have more than one issue going on in their pelvis, or one problem that may cause multi-organ symptoms. What one must realise is that these people need understanding and as much explanation as we can offer them on the current knowledge about IC, and that research is ongoing.

What are relevant questions?

IC symptoms are bladder/pelvic pain, urgency, frequency and nocturia, in **the absence** of a positive bacterial culture and cytology. IC and painful bladder syndrome share the same cluster of symptoms. Chronic urethral syndrome is an outdated term.[1] Pain distinguishes IC from overactive bladder, and vulval pain may distinguish vulvodynia from IC. Dysmenorrhoea distinguishes endometriosis from IC, although many women have endometriosis plus IC. Some women also have an overlap to irritable bowel syndrome. The Interstitial Cystitis Database Study concluded that the National Institutes of Health–National Institute of Diabetes and Digestive and Kidney Diseases (NIH-NIDDK) clinical and cystoscopic diagnostic criteria for research studies of IC were too restrictive for clinical use, because more than 60% of patients regarded by experienced clinicians as suffering from IC fail to meet the criteria.[2,3] Conversely, 90% of patients who meet the NIH-NIDDK criteria for diagnosis (glomerulations and/or ulcers) were believed by clinicians to have IC. The NIH-NIDDK criteria, though excellent for research studies, are not suitable for routine clinical diagnosis, and many clinicians are comfortable with a clinical diagnosis, although differences exist between Europe and the United States as to the benefit and place of cystoscopy and/or bladder biopsy.[4]

The questions you can ask the patient when you have calmed her down are:

● Is it painful passing urine?

● How often does she have to pass urine during the day and at night?

● Does the pain vary with her monthly cycle?

● What contraception is she using?

● Has she ever had relief using antibiotics?

● What previous investigations has she had?

What are relevant tests?

Cystoscopy

The advantages of this approach include photographic documentation of bladder inflammation (glomerulations, submucosal haemorrhages, ulcers), bladder capacity determination, exclusion of other diseases, and delineation of the degree and subtype of inflammation, if biopsies are performed. Glomerulations are not pathognomonic of IC, as glomerulations have been reported in 40% of 'normal' women undergoing tubal ligation.[5] Hydrodistension may be therapeutic, with 20%–30% of patients experiencing symptom relief for 3–6 months.

Intravesical potassium sensitivity test (Parson's Test)[6]

A dilute solution of potassium (40 mEq in 100 ml of water) is left in the bladder for five minutes. The patient then rates the degree of provocation with urgency and frequency on a scale of 0 (no provocation) to 5 (marked provocation). A positive test is defined by a change in score of 2 or more. The potassium (KCl) test has been advocated as a minimally invasive diagnostic test for IC. The intravesical potassium test fails to diagnose IC in 25% of patients with cystoscopically confirmed (NIH-NIDDK criteria) or clinically suspected IC, and gives a false positive in detrusor instability (25%), radiation cystitis (100%) and bacterial cystitis (100%). False-negative tests also occur in patients with severe disease or following treatment.

Urodynamics

Many IC patients have sensory urgency and instability, reduced bladder capacities and pain with bladder filling at low volumes. The current consensus is that urodynamic evaluation is not required for diagnosis of IC but may provide useful information regarding the differential diagnosis of painful voiding disorders and the symptoms of the overactive bladder.[7]

What treatments are available?

The various treatment options are detailed below. Often all the possible options are tried, as these patients are desperate.

- To help restore the urothelial coat, 'epithelial-coating' drugs, such as pentosan polysulphate and intravesical heparin or hyaluronic acid, have been used.

- To reduce the mast cell degranulation, antihistamines are prescribed.

- Amitriptyline may downregulate the over-sensitive neurological pathways and help with the chronic pain.

- Bladder distensions give a few months' relief.

- Diet: some people find avoiding alcohol, acidic foods, tobacco, caffeine drinks (tea, coffee, cola) and/or spicy foods improves their symptoms. Others find bottled water, rather than tap water, helpful.

- Bladder training and physiotherapy: some women find specialist physiotherapy to improve bladder capacity and pelvic floor tone helpful.

- Transcutaneous electrical nerve stimulation can be helpful for the chronic pain.

- Pregabalin may be helpful for the chronic pain.

- Botulinum toxin is being tried, but is yet to be evaluated.

Recent Developments

The urothelial surface is lined by an impermeable bladder surface mucin composed of sulphonated glycosaminoglycans and glycoproteins. Changes in this surface can allow potassium ions to go through the urothelium, depolarize sensory and motor nerves and activate mast cells.[7] Many IC sufferers have an initial proven urinary tract infection which seems to 'set off' chronic IC: it is postulated that a bacterial infection may set up an inflammatory response in the urothelium which does not settle when the infection has been cured. With these ideas in mind, treatments have been epithelial protectors and antihistamines. Urinary antiproliferative factor, found in IC, inhibits cell proliferation and impairs repair of damaged or denuded urothelium with resulting changes in the barrier function of the urothelium. Substance P, a tachykinin released by activated C-fibre afferents, is involved in nociception in the central and peripheral nervous systems and also functions as an inflammatory mediator. Substance P release results in an inflammatory cascade with mast cell activation and upregulation of adjacent nerves.[8,9] There can be autoimmune features of IC, with autoantibodies, but these may be secondary to urothelial damage. The amount of neurogenic inflammation, bladder epithelial dysfunction or mast cell activation may vary. Once the sensory nerves in the bladder are upregulated, the whole of the pelvic organs can become hypersensitive.

Evidence regarding the beneficial effects of botulinum toxin (BTX) in the treatment of pain due to IC is poor.[10] A decreased release of neuropeptides from nociceptive primary afferent nerve fibres after BTX injection has been suggested as a mechanism.

Chemical denervation caused by BTX is a reversible process as axons re-sprout within weeks to months of treatment. For this reason, repeat injection may be required to maintain the therapeutic effect.

Conclusion

IC is more prevalent than was previously thought.[11] It affects more than 800 000 women in the United States. This patient is typical as she has been symptomatic for several years and has consulted multiple physicians before diagnosis. Therefore sensitive history taking and providing an explanation and referral to a specialist are key in this patient's management. You may also wish to refer her to self-help groups for support to show that she is not alone.

Further Reading

1 Bogart LM, Berry SH, Clemens JQ. Symptoms of interstitial cystitis, painful bladder syndrome and similar diseases in women: a systematic review. *J Urol* 2007; **177**: 450–6.

2 Gillenwater JY, Wein AJ. Summary of the National Institute of Arthritis, Diabetes, Digestive and Kidney Diseases Workshop on Interstitial Cystitis, National Institutes of Health, Bethesda, Maryland, August 28–29, 1987. *J Urol* 1988; **140**: 203–6.

3 Hanno PM, Landis JR, Matthews-Cook Y, Kusek J, Nyberg L Jr. The diagnosis of interstitial cystitis revisited: lessons learned from the National Institutes of Health Interstitial Cystitis Database study. *J Urol* 1999; **161**: 553–7.

4 Sant GR, Hanno PM. Interstitial cystitis: current issues and controversies in diagnosis. *Urology* 2001; **57** (6 Suppl 1): 82–8.

5 Waxman JA, Sulak PJ, Kuehl TJ. Cystoscopic findings consistent with interstitial cystitis in normal women undergoing tubal ligation. *J Urol* 1998; **160**: 1663–7.

6 Parsons CL, Zupkas P, Parsons JK. Intravesical potassium sensitivity in patients with interstitial cystitis and urethral syndrome. *Urology* 2001; **57**: 428–32.

7 Sant GR. Etiology, pathogenesis, and diagnosis of interstitial cystitis. *Rev Urol* 2002; **4** (Suppl 1): S9–S15.

8 Marchand JE, Sant GR, Kream RM. Increased expression of substance P receptor-encoding mRNA in bladder biopsies from patients with interstitial cystitis. *Br J Urol* 1998; **81**: 224–8.

9 Theoharides TC, Kempuraj D, Sant GR. Mast cell involvement in interstitial cystitis: a review of human and experimental evidence. *Urology* 2001; **57** (Suppl 1): 47–55.

10 Sinha D, Karri K, Arunkalaivanan AS. Applications of Botulinum toxin in urogynaecology. *Eur J Obstet Gynecol Reprod Biol* 2007; **133**: 4–11.

11 Teichman JM, Parsons CL.Contemporary clinical presentation of interstitial cystitis. *Urology* 2007; **69** (Suppl 4): 41–7.

40 Urogenital Ageing – Vaginal Atrophy

Case History

A 62-year-old woman consults complaining of vaginal burning, itching and dryness. Sex has been impossible for the past six months and her husband, five years younger than herself, is starting to complain. She was unable to tolerate a speculum examination when taking of a cervical smear was attempted three months ago. She has no hot flushes and has never taken hormone replacement therapy (HRT) and does not want to take systemic oestrogens. Her last period was over ten years ago.

What is the problem?

What are the non-hormonal options?

What are the hormonal options?

How long should she be treated?

Background

What is the problem?

The problem is called urogenital atrophy and is caused by post-menopausal oestrogen deficiency.

The lower urinary and genital tracts have a common embryological origin. Oestrogen receptors and progesterone receptors are present in the vagina. Oestrogen deficiency after menopause causes atrophic changes. The vaginal mucosa becomes thinner and dry, the epithelium may become inflamed and pH increases, leading to a change in the vaginal flora. Vaginal pH rises to between pH 6.0 and pH 7.5 compared to pre-menopausal levels of pH 3.5 to pH 4.5 which help to prevent colonization with uropathogens. Colonization can lead to vaginal infection. This results in symptoms such as dyspareunia, itching, burning and dryness. The condition is common. A Dutch study of 2157 women aged 50–75 years found that overall prevalence of vaginal dryness, soreness and dyspareunia was 27%.[1] Almost half of the symptomatic women reported moderate to severe discomfort. One-third of those affected received medical care. Previous hysterectomy had no effect on the reported prevalence estimates. Hysterectomized women reported moderate to severe complaints more often than non-hysterectomized women. Smoking had no effect. A Turkish study of 500 women aged over 50 years found that 18.2% suffered from vaginal discharge and pruritus, while 23% experienced vaginal dryness.[2]

What are the non-hormonal options?

Lubricants and vaginal moisturizers are available without prescription. While being a popular first-line option, the number of published scientific trials is limited.

Lubricants usually consist of a combination of protectants and thickening agents in a water-soluble base. They are usually used as temporary measures to relieve vaginal dryness during intercourse. They therefore do not provide a long-term solution. Lubricants must be applied frequently for more continuous relief and require reapplication before sexual activity. The integrity and efficacy of condoms may be compromised by lubricants such as petroleum-based products and baby oil. This is important when condoms are used to prevent sexually transmitted infections (STIs).[3]

Moisturizers may contain a bioadhesive polycarbophil-based polymer, which attaches to mucin and epithelial cells on the vaginal wall and retains water. Moisturizers are promoted as providing long-term relief of vaginal dryness and need to be applied less frequently.[4]

What are the hormonal options?

Oestrogen-based HRT is effective in treating symptoms of vaginal atrophy in postmenopausal women. However, only a small percentage (10%) of those who would benefit from oestrogen therapy actually receive it, possibly because women are too embarrassed to seek medical help. This patient can use either systemic or local oestrogen.[5] She has elected not to take systemic therapy and the options available are low-dose natural oestrogens, such as vaginal oestriol by cream or pessary, or oestradiol by tablet or ring, which is changed every three months.[6–8] Synthetic or conjugated equine oestrogens should be avoided, as they are well absorbed from the vagina. Dienoestrol cream (a synthetic oestrogen) has been withdrawn worldwide. With the recommended low-dose oestradiol and oestriol vaginal regimens, no adverse endometrial effects should be incurred, and a progestogen need not be added for endometrial protection.[9,10] An oral oestriol tablet is available but a progestogen should be added in non-hysterectomized women.[10] A Cochrane review of vaginal oestrogens included 19 trials with 4162 women.[7] When comparing the efficacy of different oestrogenic preparations (in the form of creams, pessaries, tablets and the oestradiol-releasing vaginal ring) in relieving the symptoms of vaginal atrophy, results indicated significant findings favouring the cream, ring and tablets when compared to placebo and non-hormonal gel. Creams, pessaries, tablets and the oestradiol-releasing vaginal ring appeared to be equally effective. Fourteen trials compared safety. One trial found significant side effects following administration of cream (conjugated equine oestrogen) when compared to tablets, causing uterine bleeding, breast pain and perineal pain. Another trial found significant endometrial over-stimulation following use of the cream (conjugated equine oestrogen) when compared to the ring. Eleven studies compared acceptability to the participants by comparing comfort of product use, ease of use, overall product rating, delivery system and satisfaction. There were significant differences in adherence to treatment with the ring versus cream, favouring the ring, and also treatment acceptability favoured the ring for comfort of the product and ease of use. In the ring versus tablet group there were significant differences favouring the ring in acceptability of the treatment delivery system. There was also a significant difference in adherence to treatment in the tablets versus cream group, favouring the tablets. Overall, women appeared to favour the oestradiol-releasing vaginal ring for ease of use, comfort of product and overall satisfaction.

How long should she be treated?

It may take several months for the symptoms to improve. Examination may be avoided at the initial assessment, if she wishes, unless there has been post-coital or post-menopausal bleeding (see Case 14: Post-menopausal Bleeding). However, if her symptoms are not improved after six months it would be prudent to examine her to exclude other pathologies such as lichen sclerosus. Treatment is needed in the long term, if not lifelong, as symptoms return on cessation of treatment.

Recent Developments

Use of systemic oestrogen replacement therapy has fallen since the first publication of the Women's Health Initiative Study because of the risk of breast cancer and cardiovascular disease.[11] Thus, more women are using vaginal preparations. Treatment needs to be long-term if not lifelong as symptoms will return when it is stopped.

Conclusion

Many women suffer in silence and do not seek help. She needs to be reassured that this is a common condition and that she is not alone. Treatment may take several months to be effective and she must not expect instant results. Also, she needs to be advised of the difference between vaginal and systemic preparations in terms of potential risk.

Further Reading

1   van Geelen JM, van de Weijer PH, Arnolds HT. Urogenital symptoms and resulting discomfort in non-institutionalized Dutch women aged 50–75 years. *Int Urogynecol J Pelvic Floor Dysfunct* 2000; **11**: 9–14.

2   Oskay UY, Beji NK, Yalcin O. A study on urogenital complaints of postmenopausal women aged 50 and over. *Acta Obstet Gynecol Scand* 2005; **84**: 72–8.

3   Rosen AD, Rosen T. Study of condom integrity after brief exposure to over-the-counter vaginal preparations. *South Med J* 1999; **92**: 305–7.

4   Bygdeman M, Swahn ML. Replens versus dienoestrol cream in the symptomatic treatment of vaginal atrophy in postmenopausal women. *Maturitas* 1996; **23**: 259–63.

5   Castelo-Branco C, Cancelo MJ, Villero J, Nohales F, Juliá MD. Management of post-menopausal vaginal atrophy and atrophic vaginitis. *Maturitas* 2005; **52** (Suppl 1): S46–52.

6   Simunic V, Banovic I, Ciglar S, Jeren L, Pavicic Baldani D, Sprem M. Local estrogen treatment in patients with urogenital symptoms. *Int J Gynaecol Obstet* 2003; **82**: 187–97.

7   Suckling J, Lethaby A, Kennedy R. Local oestrogen for vaginal atrophy in postmenopausal women. *Cochrane Database Syst Rev* 2006; CD001500.

8   Nelson HD, Haney E, Humphrey L, Miller J, Nedrow A, Nicolaidis C, Vesco K, Walker M, Bougatsos C, Nygren P. Management of menopause-related symptoms. *Evid Rep Technol Assess (Summ)* 2005: 1–6.

9 Rees M, Purdie DW (eds). *Management of the Menopause: The Handbook*. London: Royal Society of Medicine Press, 2006.

10 Weiderpass E, Baron JA, Adami HO, Magnusson C, Lindgren A, Bergstrom R, Correia N, Persson I. Low-potency oestrogen and risk of endometrial cancer: a case–control study. *Lancet* 1999; **353**: 1824–8.

11 NIH State-of-the-Science Conference Statement on management of menopause-related symptoms. *NIH Consens State Sci Statements* 2005; **22**: 1–38.

Prevention and Screening

41 Cervical Cancer Prevention and Screening

Case History

A 28-year-old actress attends a consultation for contraception. She has never had a smear, as since leaving home at the age of 18 years she has never been in one place long enough to have a residential address, and has always consulted doctors for immediate problems with no proactive health planning. She is a non-smoker and uses condoms and an intrauterine contraceptive device, since in the past she has had two terminations of pregnancy.

What are the cervical screening programmes and risk factors for cervical cancer?

What are recommended screening frequencies?

What is patient care when taking a smear?

How can cervical cancer be prevented with human papillomavirus (HPV) vaccines?

Background

What are the cervical screening programmes and risk factors for cervical cancer?

Worldwide, about 500 000 cases of cervical cancer are estimated to occur each year,[1] over 80% of which occur in developing countries where neither population-based routine

Table 41.1 Risk factors for cervical cancer
● Human papillomavirus is the essential causative factor
● Smoking – which reduces immunity
● Immunosuppression – including human immunodeficiency virus (HIV) infection
● High parity, use of combined oral contraception and co-infection with sexually transmitted infections are also factors, although less important

screening (e.g. Papanicolaou smear test) nor optimal treatment are available. Risk factors for cervical cancer are detailed in Table 41.1.

Screening is, by definition, the examination of asymptomatic individuals in an attempt to identify pre-invasive disease, early disease or the risk factors for a disease. Cervical screening programmes vary worldwide and in some countries there are none. In England, where there is a cervical screening programme, cervical cancer incidence fell by 42% between 1988 and 1997 in England and Wales.[2] An analysis of trends in mortality from cervical cancer before and after cervical screening was introduced in England suggests that up to 4500 lives are saved each year as a result of screening.[3] Nevertheless, 927 deaths from invasive cervical cancer were registered in 2002.

What are recommended screening frequencies?

Controversy remains over the most appropriate screening interval. Annual screening is common in the United States and five-yearly screening is offered in some European countries. In England, the current recommendations comprise a first invitation at 25 years of age, interval screening three-yearly from age 25–49, and five-yearly from age 50–64 years. In Scotland, the recommendations differ in that all women over the age of 20 years are invited every three years until the age of 60 years. By screening every five years, the incidence of the disease falls by 84%. Reducing the screening interval to three-yearly leads to a further reduction in incidence of cervical cancer of 91%. Women who have never been sexually active have an extremely low chance of developing cervical cancer, and although they will be invited for cervical screening they can choose to decline. Women who have had a subtotal hysterectomy (i.e. have the cervix retained at surgery) must continue to have routine smears: sometimes the women themselves do not realise that they still need a smear.

What is patient care when taking a smear?

The questions you need to ask are detailed in Table 41.2.

The most common error in taking a smear is failing to take an adequate sample from the squamocolumnar junction, the area where neoplastic change occurs. In nulliparous women and in women beyond the menopause, the squamocolumnar junction may be well within the cervical canal and it is not always possible to sample this area.

Swift referral to colposcopy is required for cervical carcinoma, severe dyskaryosis or moderate dyskaryosis. Women with a mild or borderline smear should have a repeat smear in six months' time with colposcopy referral if this is again abnormal.

Doctors should be clear about the facilities for investigation and treatment available locally. Colposcopic examination and treatment services are widely available in the

Table 41.2 Questions to be asked before taking a smear
● When was your last smear?
● Have you ever had a sexually transmitted disease?
● Have you ever had bleeding mid-cycle or after sex?
● Have you ever been treated in the past for an abnormal smear?
● Are you happy with your present contraception?

United Kingdom and the traditional cone biopsy will be avoided in the vast majority of women with abnormal smears. Local ablative treatments include excision by loop diathermy, cold coagulation and laser vaporization.[4]

How can cervical cancer be prevented with human papillomavirus (HPV) vaccines?

The role of HPV in cervical dysplasia and neoplasia has been recognized since the 1970s. Several subtypes of this virus have been implicated in the aetiology of cervical cancer.[1,3] The most relevant of these are HPV types 16 and 18 which are 'highly oncogenic' and account for 70% of all cervical cancers. HPV types 6 and 11 cause genital warts but not cervical disease and there is no need, therefore, to screen women with warts more frequently.

Around 60% of women with mild dyskaryosis reported on cervical cytology will spontaneously clear the virus and subsequent smears will be normal. Approximately 10% of those with mild dyskaryosis will, however, progress to having severe dyskaryosis within 2–4 years.[5] It is not currently possible to distinguish these two groups. Although it is possible to test for HPV types, this is neither cost-effective nor widely available.

HPV vaccines

Two vaccines against HPV have been developed (see Case 45: Cervical Cancer).[1,6] One (Gardasil®) is now licensed for girls and women aged 9–26 years, and the other (Cervarix™) was licensed in the UK in November 2007. These vaccines, prepared from the virus-like particles of the major coat or capsid protein L1 of HPV, induce neutralizing antibodies to the oncogenic subtypes. Cervarix™ is a bivalent vaccine against HPV types 16 and 18 and Gardasil® is a quadrivalent vaccine against HPV types 6, 11, 16 and 18, which thus also protects against genital warts. In Phase III trials of both vaccines there was 100% efficacy against development of HPV type 16/18-associated cervical intraepithelial neoplasia (CIN) 2/3.[7,8] As yet, the duration of protection of these vaccines is unknown, as is whether booster immunization will be required. There is some evidence of cross-protection against other HPV types which are less oncogenic.

Recent Developments

1   Liquid-based cytology (LBC) is replacing the classical smear test as a method of screening. It involves a plastic broom device instead of a wooden spatula to take the smear and is suitable for automated screening. Introduction of the technique varies worldwide. LBC also allows testing for HPV and molecular markers of

cervical neoplasia such as p16INK4a, minichromosome maintenance proteins 2, 4 and 5, and cyclin D1.[10] HPV testing and surrogate molecular markers of HPV-mediated dysplasia and carcinoma are likely to have increasingly important roles for the triage of patients with low-grade cervical cytologic abnormalities and for the reduction of risk of false-negative cytology test results.

2   Guidance as to who should receive which HPV vaccination is currently awaited. Ideally, young people should be vaccinated prior to becoming sexually active. However, vaccination could provide protection for those who are already sexually active but have not been exposed to the specific HPV types. The debate as to which vaccine should be recommended will continue. There are arguments in favour of vaccinating boys with the quadrivalent vaccine to attempt to eradicate genital warts and girls with the bivalent vaccine which may provide longer protection against HPV types 16 and 18. Cervical screening will remain necessary for many years to come as it is unlikely that all women will be vaccinated, and even those who are will remain vulnerable to infection with other HPV types which may cause abnormalities. The American Cancer Society has produced a guideline for vaccine use (Table 41.3).[9]

Table 41.3 American Cancer Society (ACS) Guideline for HPV vaccine use to prevent cervical cancer and its precursors

- Routine HPV vaccination is recommended for females aged 11 to 12 years.
- Females as young as age 9 years may receive HPV vaccination.
- HPV vaccination is also recommended for females aged 13 to 18 years to catch up missed vaccine or complete the vaccination series.
- There are currently insufficient data to recommend for or against universal vaccination of females aged 19 to 26 years in the general population. A decision about whether a woman aged 19 to 26 years should receive the vaccine should be based on an informed discussion between the woman and her healthcare provider regarding her risk of previous HPV exposure and potential benefit from vaccination. Ideally, the vaccine should be administered prior to potential exposure to genital HPV through sexual intercourse because the potential benefit is likely to diminish with increasing number of lifetime sexual partners.
- HPV vaccination is not currently recommended for women over age 26 years or for males.
- Screening for CIN and cancer should continue in both vaccinated and unvaccinated women according to current ACS early detection guidelines.

Source: Saslow *et al.* 2007.[9]

Conclusion

This woman has never had a cervical smear and it is thus essential that she is told about the effectiveness of cervical screening in reducing the numbers of invasive cancers.

Further Reading

1   World Health Organization. Vaccinating against cervical cancer. *Bull World Health Organ* 2007; **85**: 89–90.

2 Cancer Research UK, June 2006. www.cancerresearchuk.org (accessed 02 10 07)

3 Lowndes CM, Gill ON. Cervical cancer, human papillomavirus, and vaccination. *BMJ* 2005; **331**: 915–16.

4 Harper C. Cervical cytology and colposcopy. In: Rees M, Hope S (eds). *Specialist Training in Gynaecology*. Edinburgh: Elsevier Mosby, 2005; 111–27.

5 Kjaer S, Hogdall E, Frederiksen K, Munk C, van den Brule A, Svare E, Meijer C, Lorincz A, Iftner T. The absolute risk of cervical abnormalities in high-risk human papillomavirus-positive, cytologically normal women over a 10-year period. *Cancer Res* 2006; **66**: 10630–6.

6 Quilliam S. Cervical cancer and the human papillomavirus vaccine. *J Fam Plann Reprod Health Care* 2006; **32**: 119–20.

7 Villa LL, Costa RL, Petta CA, Andrade RP, Paavonen J, Iversen OE, Olsson SE, Hoye J, Steinwall M, Riis-Johannessen G, Andersson-Ellstrom A, Elfgren K, Krogh G, Lehtinen M, Malm C, Tamms GM, Giacoletti K, Lupinacci L, Railkar R, Taddeo FJ, Bryan J, Esser MT, Sings HL, Saah AJ, Barr E. High sustained efficacy of a prophylactic quadrivalent human papillomavirus types 6/11/16/18 L1 virus-like particle vaccine through 5 years of follow-up. *Br J Cancer* 2006; **95**: 1459–66.

8 Harper DM, Franco EL, Wheeler CM, Moscicki AB, Romanowski B, Roteli-Martins CM, Jenkins D, Schuind A, Costa Clemens SA, Dubin G; HPV Vaccine Study group. Sustained efficacy up to 4.5 years of a bivalent L1 virus-like particle vaccine against human papillomavirus types 16 and 18: follow-up from a randomised control. *Lancet* 2006; **367**: 1247–55.

9 Saslow D, Castle PE, Cox JT, Davey DD, Einstein MH, Ferris DG, Goldie SJ, Harper DM, Kinney W, Moscicki AB, Noller KL, Wheeler CM, Ades T, Andrews KS, Doroshenk MK, Kahn KG, Schmidt C, Shafey O, Smith RA, Partridge EE; Gynecologic Cancer Advisory Group, Garcia F. American Cancer Society Guideline for human papillomavirus (HPV) vaccine use to prevent cervical cancer and its precursors. *CA Cancer J Clin* 2007; **57**: 7–28.

10 Dehn D, Torkko KC, Shroyer KR. Human papillomavirus testing and molecular markers of cervical dysplasia and carcinoma. *Cancer* 2007; **111**: 1–14.

42 Breast Cancer Screening in Normal and High-risk Populations

Case History

A 43-year-old woman who has been taking combined hormone replacement therapy (HRT) since the age of 38 for premature ovarian failure is concerned about breast cancer because her sister and a cousin have recently been diagnosed with breast cancer in their early 50s. Should she have mammography?

Is she at high risk of breast cancer?

What mammographic screening should be offered?

Does HRT affect mammography?

Background

Is she at high risk of breast cancer?

Concern about familial breast cancer is a common problem. In the United Kingdom (UK), the National Institute for Clinical Excellence (NICE) has produced clinical guidance for the classification and care of women at risk of familial breast cancer and the need for mammograms (Table 42.1).[1]

This woman is not at increased risk of breast cancer since she has only one first-degree and one third-degree relative (her cousin) diagnosed with breast cancer after the age of 50 years. If she had other relatives with breast cancer increasing her risk, the following would be suggested. Current recommendations in the UK for mammographic surveillance of women at moderate risk or greater are that:

● It should not be available for women younger than 30 years

● It should only be performed as part of a research study or nationally approved and audited service for those aged 30–39 years

● It should be performed annually for women aged 40–49 years

● It should be performed every three years as part of the National Health Service Breast Screening Programme for women aged ≥50 years.[2]

What mammographic screening should be offered?

Mammography is the preferred method for screening since the role of magnetic resonance imaging (MRI) and ultrasound is uncertain. MRI is more sensitive than mammog-

Table 42.1 Clinical guidance for the classification and care of women at risk of familial breast cancer

Women likely to be at moderate risk (i.e. lifetime risk between 17% and less than 30%)
- One 1st degree relative diagnosed before age 40 years
- One 1st degree relative and one 2nd degree relative diagnosed after average age of 50 years
- Two 1st degree relatives diagnosed after average age of 50 years

Women likely to be at more than moderate risk (i.e. lifetime risk of more than 30%)
Female breast cancer only
- One 1st degree relative and one 2nd degree relative diagnosed before average age of 50 years
- Two 1st degree relatives diagnosed before average age of 50 years
- Three or more 1st or 2nd degree relatives diagnosed at any age

Male breast cancer
- 1st degree male relative diagnosed at any age

Bilateral breast cancer (cancer in both breasts)
- One 1st degree relative where the first primary cancer diagnosed before age 50 years

Breast and ovarian cancer
- One 1st or 2nd degree relative with ovarian cancer at any age and one 1st or 2nd degree relative with breast cancer at any age (one should be a 1st degree relative)

1st degree relative: mother, father, daughter, son, sister, brother;
2nd degree relative: grandparents, grandchildren, aunt, uncle, niece, nephew, half sister, half brother;
3rd degree relative: great grandparents, great grandchildren, great aunt, great uncle, first cousin, grand nephew, grand niece;
Source: adapted from NICE, 2004 (Familial breast cancer; quick reference guide).[1]

raphy (fewer false negatives), but its specificity is lower (more false positives).[3] In the UK, the National Institute for Health and Clinical Excellence recommends the use of MRI for screening in women aged under 50 with familial breast cancer.[1] Mammography screening programmes vary throughout the world. In the UK all women aged 50–70 years are invited to have a mammogram every three years. This screening is also offered to older women but they need to initiate the mammogram.

Does HRT affect mammography?

There is now extensive evidence that a mammographic density is a risk factor for breast cancer, independent of other risk factors.[4] Observational studies show that taking HRT is associated with an increase in breast density on mammography. However, randomized placebo-controlled trials (the Women's Health Initiative [WHI] and Progestin Estrogen–Progestin Intervention [PEPI] studies) have shown that not all HRT regimens have this effect.[5–8] Unopposed oestrogen (that is, conjugated equine oestrogen) does not seem to induce any increase in density, whereas combined therapy (both cyclical and continuous combined) does, on average, in one in four women who take it. Also, if any increase in density occurs, it takes place within the first year of exposure, and no evidence shows that duration of use influences this effect. The PEPI and WHI trials additionally reported that the individual degree of increase in density associated with exposure to combined HRT is in the order of 3%–6%. Currently, published data from placebo-controlled, randomized trials that evaluated the effect of unopposed oestradiol on mammographic density and observational studies are inconsistent. Thus, breast density on mammography is unlikely to be affected by current use of HRT in most women. Breast density may be reduced in women taking tibolone.[9]

Withdrawal of HRT before mammography has been reported to result in regression of increases in density associated with HRT sufficient to enable more accurate film reading.[10] While this effect has not been subject to controlled evaluation, it may occur in as little as two weeks.

By increasing breast density, combined HRT can reduce the sensitivity and specificity of mammography. This would be expected to result in an increase in interval cancers (that is, cancers missed during screening because of decreased sensitivity) and has been reported in observational studies such as the Million Women study. However, interval cancers diagnosed in women who take HRT have not been reported to have more adverse prognostic features.

Recent Developments

1   No evidence supports routine mammographic examination of the breasts in women about to start HRT. There is also no evidence to suggest that women on HRT require mammography more frequently than the national screening programmes, such as that offered in the UK. Also women with premature menopause taking HRT do not need to have extra mammograms outside screening programmes.

2   There is also no evidence that women taking HRT before the age of 50 increase their risk of breast cancer to more than that found in normally menstruating women.[11]

Conclusion

It is important that this patient is reassured. The need for taking HRT until the average age of the natural menopause should be reiterated (see Case 12: Premature Menopause). However, she should be advised that if her family history changes she should consult again.

Further Reading

1   National Institute for Health and Clinical Excellence (NICE). *Familial breast cancer: the classification and care of women at risk of familial breast cancer in primary, secondary and tertiary care.* NICE Clinical Guideline No. 41. London: NICE, 2004 (updated 2006). Available at: http://guidance.nice.org.uk/cg41/?c=91496 (accessed 18 09 07)

2   NHS Breast Screening Programme (NHSBSP). www.cancerscreening.nhs.uk/breastscreen (accessed 18 09 07)

3   Leach MO, Boggis CR, Dixon AK, Easton DF, Eeles RA, Evans DG, Gilbert FJ, Griebsch I, Hoff RJ, Kessar P, Lakhani SR, Moss SM, Nerurkar A, Padhani AR, Pointon LJ, Thompson D, Warren RM; MARIBS study group. Screening with magnetic resonance imaging and mammography of a UK population at high familial risk of breast cancer: a prospective multicentre cohort study (MARIBS). *Lancet* 2005; **365**: 1769–78.

4 Boyd NF, Guo H, Martin LJ, Sun L, Stone J, Fishell E, Jong RA, Hislop G, Chiarelli A, Minkin S, Yaffe MJ. Mammographic density and the risk and detection of breast cancer. *N Engl J Med* 2007; **356**: 227–36.

5 Chlebowski RT, Hendrix SL, Langer RD, Stefanick ML, Gass M, Lane D, Rodabough RJ, Gilligan MA, Cyr MG, Thomson CA, Khandekar J, Petrovitch H, McTiernan A; WHI Investigators. Influence of estrogen plus progestin on breast cancer and mammography in healthy postmenopausal women: the Women's Health Initiative Randomized Trial. *JAMA* 2003; **289**: 3243–53.

6 McTiernan A, Martin CF, Peck JD, Aragaki AK, Chlebowski RT, Pisano ED, Wang CY, Brunner RL, Johnson KC, Manson JE, Lewis CE, Kotchen JM, Hulka BS; Women's Health Initiative Mammogram Density Study Investigators. Estrogen-plus-progestin use and mammographic density in postmenopausal women: women's health initiative randomized trial. *J Natl Cancer Inst* 2005; **97**: 1366–76.

7 Greendale GA, Reboussin BA, Sie A, Singh HR, Olson LK, Gatewood O, Bassett LW, Wasilauskas C, Bush T, Barrett-Connor E. Effects of estrogen and estrogen–progestin on mammographic parenchymal density. Postmenopausal Estrogen/Progestin Interventions (PEPI) Investigators. *Ann Intern Med* 1999; **130**: 262–9.

8 Greendale GA, Reboussin BA, Slone S, Wasilauskas C, Pike MC, Ursin G. Postmenopausal hormone therapy and change in mammographic density. *J Natl Cancer Inst* 2003; **95**: 30–7.

9 von Schoultz B. The effects of tibolone and oestrogen-based HT on breast cell proliferation and mammographic density. *Maturitas* 2004; **49**: S16–21.

10 Colacurci N, Fornaro F, De Franciscis P, Mele D, Palermo M, del Vecchio W. Effects of a short-term suspension of hormone replacement therapy on mammographic density. *Fertil Steril* 2001; **76**: 451–5.

11 Ewertz M, Mellemkjaer L, Poulsen AH, Friis S, Sorensen HT, Pedersen L, McLaughlin JK, Olsen JH. Hormone use for menopausal symptoms and risk of breast cancer. A Danish cohort study. *Br J Cancer* 2005; **92**: 1293–7.

43 Ovarian Cancer Screening in Normal and High-risk Populations

Case History

A 35-year-old woman's mother died at age 49 years from epithelial ovarian cancer. There is no other family history of cancer. She wants to be counselled with regard to ovarian cancer screening.

Who should be screened, and what constitutes high risk?

What is the most appropriate screening method?

At what age should screening commence, and what is the most appropriate screening interval?

Is screening the best way to manage risk, and what are the alternatives?

Background

Who should be screened, and what constitutes high risk?

Ovarian cancer is responsible for more deaths per year in the industrialized world than cervical and endometrial cancer combined. The poor prognosis for women with ovarian cancer is related to the fact that the disease is usually diagnosed at an advanced stage. By the time the patient develops symptoms and is investigated, the disease has usually progressed and chances of cure are minimal. Therefore great interest exists in early detection of ovarian cancer through screening in asymptomatic women.

Screening for ovarian cancer, however, is hampered by (a) the low incidence of ovarian cancer in the general population, (b) the lack of identification of an ovarian cancer precursor lesion and pre-clinical asymptomatic disease, and (c) the lack of sufficient sensitivity and specificity of established screening tests (serum CA125 measurement and transvaginal ultrasound scan [TVS]).

Large randomized clinical trials (Prostate, Lung, Colorectal and Ovarian Screening Trial; United Kingdom Collaborative Trial of Ovarian Cancer Screening) have been initiated to evaluate whether ovarian cancer screening in the general population by serum CA125 measurement and transvaginal ultrasound scan can reduce mortality. These trials might provide the standards for screening efficacy but will not be completed for several years.[1,2] As this evidence is not available, screening for ovarian cancer in the general population is not recommended by any medical organization at this time.[3]

Table 43.1 Women at moderate risk of developing ovarian cancer
● One first- or second-degree relative diagnosed with ovarian cancer (provided that family is not of Ashkenazi Jewish ancestry and does not have additional cases of breast cancer)
● Two first- or second-degree relatives with ovarian cancer on different sides of the family

Similarly, screening for women at only moderately increased risk of developing ovarian cancer (Table 43.1) is usually not justified. For those women, the lifetime risk of ovarian cancer is between 1 in 100 and 1 in 30. This risk is no more than three times the population average. Those women should be advised to visit their general practitioner promptly with any health changes.[4]

Women with ovarian cancer risk that is considerably above the average (Table 43.2) might benefit from screening. These women have a lifetime risk of ovarian cancer between 1 in 30 and 1 in 3. This risk is more than three times the population average. Individual risk might even be higher if tests are positive for a gene mutation.[4] *BRCA1* mutation carriers have a lifetime risk of ovarian cancer of up to 60%; *BRCA2* mutation carriers a risk of up to 40%. The lifetime risk of ovarian cancer for a woman with hereditary non-polyposis colorectal cancer is about 10%.

A woman with a high-risk family history but without known gene mutation should be advised about her potential risk of developing ovarian cancer and possibly other cancers such as of the breast. A referral to a specialist familial cancer centre should be made if the woman wishes to clarify her genetic risk. However, it is also important to inform the woman that the majority of high-risk individuals will not develop ovarian cancer.[4]

Table 43.2 Women at high risk of developing ovarian cancer
● Two first- or second-degree relatives on the same side of the family diagnosed with epithelial ovarian cancer (especially if additional relatives with breast cancer occur)
● One first-degree relative diagnosed with ovarian cancer in a family of Ashkenazi Jewish ancestry
● One relative with ovarian cancer at any age and one with breast cancer before the age of 50 years, where the women are first- or second-degree relatives of each other
● Three or more first- or second-degree relatives on the same side of the family diagnosed with any cancers associated with hereditary non-polyposis colorectal cancer.

What is the most appropriate screening method?

While screening of women at high risk may be appropriate, they should be made aware of the current limitations of surveillance. It has to be emphasized that there is no definitive evidence about whether surveillance will reduce mortality. An appropriate screening programme for women with high risk of ovarian cancer includes a transvaginal ultrasound scan, with or without colour Doppler imaging, in combination with serum CA125 measurements.[5] This combined approach has been shown to be more successful than using either test alone and has a positive predictive value of about 10%.[6] Therefore, an average of ten surgical procedures for each detected ovarian cancer have to be performed.

All women undergoing screening have to be aware of the significant false-positive rate of ovarian cancer screening, which is highest in pre-menopausal women.

At what age should screening commence, and what is the most appropriate screening interval?

Screening with ultrasound scan and serum CA125 measurement for high-risk women should commence at age 35 years or at least five years earlier than the age at diagnosis of the youngest ovarian cancer case in the family. Annual surveillance is usually recommended, although the optimal screening interval is not known. Consideration, however, should be given to the psychological effects that screening may have if the intervals are short, with particular reference to the likelihood of a false-positive screening result in pre-menopausal women.

Is screening the best way to manage risk, and what are the alternatives?

For women who are not eligible for screening because their ovarian cancer risk is average or only moderately increased, there is convincing evidence that the use of the combined oral contraceptive (COC) pill has a significant protective effect against ovarian cancer. Women who have ever used the oral contraceptive pill have a 50% risk reduction compared to women who have never used it. The benefit increases with duration of use and extends well beyond the period of use. There is approximately 6% reduction of risk for each year of use of the pill.[7] Overall, the current evidence suggests a similar risk reduction for ovarian cancer in women who use the oral contraceptive pill and who are carriers of a mutation in the *BRCA1* or *BRCA2* genes.[7]

Women who are at high risk for ovarian cancer and have completed their families should be counselled about risk-reducing surgery (e.g. a prophylactic salpingo-oophorectomy). Women with documented *BRCA1* or *BRCA2* mutations who undergo risk-reducing salpingo-oophorectomy have a 80%–96% reduction in the risk of ovarian and fallopian tube cancer (see Case 50: Prophylactic Salpingo-oophorectomy).[8,9]

Recent Developments

In an effort to develop an early detection test suitable for ovarian cancer screening, new research in the area of proteomics has occurred. The aim is to identify proteins and peptides that have different expression patterns characteristic of cancerous and non-cancerous states. Large numbers of blood protein levels are compared using sophisticated pattern-recognition algorithms to discover unique 'fingerprints' associated with early ovarian cancer. An initial study by a collaborative proteomics team of the United States Food and Drug Administration (FDA) and National Institutes of Health – National Cancer Institute (NCI), applying surface-enhanced laser desorption and ionization technology, reported a very high sensitivity (100%) and specificity (95%) by analyzing the pattern of proteins expressed in sera from ovarian cancer patients and healthy individuals. The proteomic pattern completely discriminated cancer from non-cancer.[10] Based on these findings, a test was developed and marketed under the brand name OvaCheck™ (Correlogic Systems Inc., Bethesda, MD). However, the reliability and reproducibility of this test has been questioned.[11] Consequently, the FDA declared OvaCheck™ to be a medical device[12] which has to be validated by well-designed, large-population, randomized, controlled clinical trials in relation to patient outcomes, patient morbidity and mortality. Therefore, as results of these studies are pending, the role of OvaCheck™ in the screening of ovarian cancer remains unknown. However, despite initial difficulties, it is very likely that some form of effective screening for ovarian cancer is going to emerge from further developments of proteomic testing.

Conclusion

This patient is at moderately increased risk since she only has one first-degree relative with ovarian cancer and does not have additional cases of breast cancer. Nor is she of Ashkenazi Jewish ancestry. Thus, screening is not justified at present. However, she should be advised to consult again should her family history change.

Further Reading

1 Prorok PC, Andriole GL, Bresalier RS, Buys SS, Chia D, Crawford ED, Fogel R, Gelmann EP, Gilbert F, Hasson MA, Hayes RB, Johnson CC, Mandel JS, Oberman A, O'Brien B, Oken MM, Rafla S, Reding D, Rutt W, Weissfeld JL, Yokochi L, Gohagan JK. Design of the Prostate, Lung, Colorectal and Ovarian (PLCO) Cancer Screening Trial. *Control Clin Trials* 2000; **21**: 273S–309S.

2 Sharma A, Menon U. Screening for gynaecological cancers. *Eur J Surg Oncol* 2006; **32**: 818–24.

3 US Preventive Services Task Force. Screening for ovarian cancer: recommendation statement. US Preventive Services Task Force. *Am Fam Physician* 2005; **71**: 759–62.

4 National Breast Cancer Centre (NBCC), Australia. *Advice about familial aspects of breast cancer and ovarian cancer: a guide for health professionals.* Camperdown, NSW: NBCC, 2006. www.nbcc.org.au/bestpractice/ (accessed 20 09 07)

5 Pichert G, Bolliger B, Buser K, Pagani O. Evidence-based management options for women at increased breast/ovarian cancer risk. *Ann Oncol* 2003; **14**: 9–19.

6 Bosse K, Rhiem K, Wappenschmidt B, Hellmich M, Madeja M, Ortmann M, Mallmann P, Schmutzler R. Screening for ovarian cancer by transvaginal ultrasound and serum CA125 measurement in women with a familial predisposition: a prospective cohort study. *Gynecol Oncol* 2006; **103**: 1077–82.

7 McGuire V, Felberg A, Mills M, Ostrow KL, DiCioccio R, John EM, West DW, Whittemore AS. Relation of contraceptive and reproductive history to ovarian cancer risk in carriers and noncarriers of *BRCA1* gene mutations *Am J Epidemiol* 2004; **160**: 613–18.

8 Finch A, Beiner M, Lubinski J, Lynch HT, Moller P, Rosen B, Murphy J, Ghadirian P, Friedman E, Foulkes WD, Kim-Sing C, Wagner T, Tung N, Couch F, Stoppa-Lyonnet D, Ainsworth P, Daly M, Pasini B, Gershoni-Baruch R, Eng C, Olopade OI, McLennan J, Karlan B, Weitzel J, Sun P, Narod SA. Salpingo-oophorectomy and the risk of ovarian, fallopian tube, and peritoneal cancers in women with a *BRCA1* or *BRCA2* mutation. *JAMA* 2006; **296**: 185–92.

9 Rebbeck TR, Lynch HT, Neuhausen SL, Narod SA, Van't Veer L, Garber JE, Evans G, Isaacs C, Daly MB, Matloff E, Olopade OI, Weber BL. Prophylactic oophorectomy in carriers of *BRCA1* or *BRCA2* mutations. *N Engl J Med* 2002; **346**: 1616–22.

10 Petricoin EF, Ardekani AM, Hitt BA, Levine PJ, Fusaro VA, Steinberg SM, Mills GB, Simone C, Fishman DA, Kohn EC, Liotta LA. Use of proteomic patterns in serum to identify ovarian cancer. *Lancet* 2002; **359**: 572–7.

11 Check E. Proteomics and cancer: running before we can walk? *Nature* 2004; **429**: 496–7.

12 US Food and Drug Administration. Center for Devices and Radiological Health. Office of In Vitro Diagnostic Device Evaluation and Safety. Letter to Correlogic Systems, Inc. July 12, 2004. www.fda.gov/cdrh/oivd/letters/071204-correlogic.html (accessed 20 09 07)

PROBLEM

44 Osteoporosis Screening

Case History

A woman seeks your advice. She is peri-menopausal, 49 years old and getting hot flushes, which are tolerable. She did not have any menstrual periods for the six years she was at university and in the cross-country orienteering team. Two of her cousins have breast cancer. Her mother died post-operatively after a fractured neck of femur at age 64 years, sustained slipping in the supermarket. Her children are 10 and 14 years old. She wants to remain fit and healthy 'to look after my grandchildren, so I don't want breast cancer or osteoporosis!'

What is osteoporosis?

What should you ask and what tests should you do?

What can she do to reduce her risk?

Background

What is osteoporosis?

Osteoporosis is a major problem with one in three women aged over 50 years and one in twelve men having one or more osteoporotic fracture.[1] The classic osteoporotic fractures are hip, vertebral and wrist fractures. The cost of osteoporotic fracture is high. For

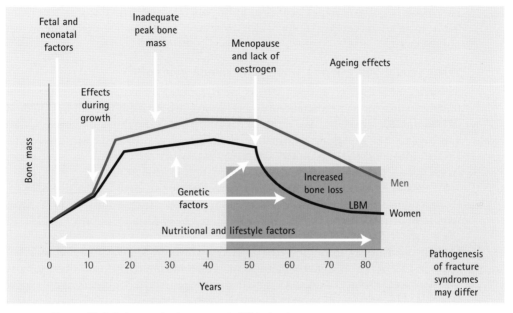

Figure 44.1 Pathogenesis of osteoporosis: LBM = low bone mass.

example, the cost for hip fractures worldwide is estimated to be US $34 800 million in 1990 and to reach $131 500 million in 2050.[2] The lifetime risk in the United States for a hip, spine or forearm fracture at the age of 50 years has been estimated to be 40% in women and 13% in men.[3] In Sweden, the corresponding figures are 46% for women and 22% for men. Women need to understand the multifactorial aetiology of osteoporosis in order to maximize their bone strength in the post-menopausal period (Figure 44.1).

Osteoporosis is defined in a National Institutes of Health consensus statement as 'a skeletal disorder characterized by compromised bone strength predisposing to an increased risk of fracture'.[4] Bone strength reflects the integration of two main features: bone density and bone quality. Bone density is expressed as grams of mineral per area or volume and, in any given individual, is determined by peak bone mass and amount of bone loss. Bone quality refers to architecture, turnover, damage accumulation (for example, microfractures) and mineralization.

On the basis of the measurement of bone mineral density (BMD) (Table 44.1), the World Health Organization's definitions, applied to post-menopausal women, result in

Table 44.1 Definitions of osteoporosis according to the World Health Organization	
Description	Definition
Normal	A person has a BMD value between −1 SD and +1 SD of the young adult mean (T-score −1 to +1)
Osteopenia	A person has a BMD reduced between −1 and −2.5 SD from the young adult mean (T-score −1 to −2.5)
Osteoporosis	A person has a BMD reduced by equal to or more than −2.5 SD from the young adult mean (T-score −2.5 or lower)

30% of this population being classified as having osteoporosis.[5] The T-score is that number of standard deviations (SD) by which the bone in question differs from the young, normal mean.

What should you ask and what tests should you do?

Screening and advice on osteoporosis needs to be holistic. Understand the reasons about the fears, concerns and expectations of that woman. This patient has had her children late, so they are still young. She needs to maximize her fitness through the menopause and beyond. She is seeking information and might find dedicated charities like the United Kingdom (UK) National Osteoporosis Society very useful as a resource (www.nos.org.uk), as they have excellent information accessible to all.

General agreement is that population screening for osteoporosis is not advised. However, since this woman's mother had a fractured neck of femur and the patient had a significant period of secondary amenorrhoea, it may be prudent to measure her BMD to assess if she is at risk or not (Table 44.2).

Dual-energy X-ray absorptiometry (DEXA) is an X-ray–based system that uses two different energies to differentiate between soft tissue and bone. The main sites for measurement are the spine (L1 or L2–L4) and the hip. Peripheral DEXA systems are also now available to measure the forearm or calcaneus and may be considered to be a risk-assessment tool. They cannot replace hip DEXA, however, for the formal diagnosis of osteoporosis.

Table 44.2 Risk factors for osteoporosis

- Age (>65 years)
- Family history of fracture (particularly a first-degree relative with hip fracture)
- Previous fragility fracture (a fall from standing height or less in a >45-year-old)
- Oral glucocorticoid therapy
- Current smoking
- Alcohol intake >3 units/day
- Rheumatoid arthritis
- Immobility (paralysis for any reason)
- Falls
- Body mass index <19 kg/m²
- Premature menopause
- Secondary amenorrhoea
- Untreated hypogonadism
- Malabsorption
- Chronic liver disease
- Chronic renal disease
- Other endocrine disease (thyroid, parathyroid)
- Medication (aromatase inhibitors, androgen deprivation therapy)

What can she do to reduce her risk?

If the woman is peri-menopausal without any other risk factors, such as glucocorticoid use, and her BMD is normal, she can be reassured and reassessed at the age of 65–70 years.[6,7] A decade ago she might have been offered hormone replacement therapy to help maintain bone density, but regulatory bodies such as those in the UK no longer recommend it due to the long-term risks of breast cancer.[8] She needs the following lifestyle advice:[9]

1. Stop smoking

Smoking kills by increasing the risks of various cancers and by thromboembolic events. Before it does this, it also thins the bones, although the mechanism is uncertain.

2. Reduce alcohol

The Million Women study[10] showed that an alcohol intake >3 units/day doubles the risk of breast cancer. Middle-aged women need to know this. It is also an independent risk factor for osteoporosis.

3. Modest weight-bearing exercise

The positive message for 20 minutes weight-bearing exercise three times a week is already known for improving cardiovascular strength, lowering blood pressure and improving mood. It is also good for bones. Excessive, compulsive exercising induces secondary amenorrhoea and is bad for bones. Women need to know that swimming, whilst good for the cardiovascular system, is useless for strengthening bones as the exercise needs to be against gravity.

4. Healthy diet

Most people in the UK by the end of February are vitamin D deficient; the benefit of going outside to exercise maximizes sun exposure during the winter. People in residential old people's homes and the housebound are vitamin D deficient all year round as they

Table 44.3 Calcium content of some foods	
Food	Calcium content (mg)
Full-fat milk (250 ml)	295
Semi-skimmed milk (250 ml)	300
Skimmed milk (250 ml)	305
Low-fat yogurt (100 g)	150
Cheddar cheese (50 g)	360
Boiled spinach (100 g)	159
Brazil nuts (100 g)	170
Tinned salmon (100 g)	93
Tofu (100 g)	480

Source: Rees and Purdie (eds) 2006 (with permission).[11]

never go out. Some people do not take enough calcium in their diet via milk and dairy produce, and require about 1000 mg/day before the menopause and 1500 mg/day thereafter (Table 44.3).[11]

Recent Developments

Osteoporosis is operationally defined in terms of bone mineral density. The clinical development of pharmaceutical agents has focused on the selection of patients on the basis of low BMD for inclusion into trials of efficacy. As a consequence, guidance on therapeutic intervention has also emphasized the assessment of BMD. However, the risk of fracture is multifactorial and many independent clinical risk factors have been identified that contribute to risk over and above that reflected by BMD. Models have been developed based on population studies to provide the basis for the integrated use of validated clinical risk factors in men and women to aid in fracture risk prediction.[12] The combination of clinical risk factors and BMD will provide higher specificity and sensitivity than either alone and this is of importance in deciding optimal use for prevention of osteoporosis with pharmaceutical agents.

Conclusion

Management of this patient will depend on her BMD. Even if it is normal, she should be advised to reduce her risk with the lifestyle measures discussed above. Her calcium intake should be assessed and, if deficient, she should take a supplement.

Further Reading

1 National Osteoporosis Society. What is osteoporosis? www.nos.org.uk/about.htm

2 Johnell O. The socioeconomic burden of fractures: today and in the 21st century. *Am J Med* 1997; **103**: 20S–25S.

3 Johnell O, Kanis J. Epidemiology of osteoporotic fractures. *Osteoporos Int* 2005; **16** (Suppl 2): S3–7.

4 NIH Consensus Development Panel on Osteoporosis Prevention, Diagnosis, and Therapy. Osteoporosis prevention, diagnosis, and therapy. *JAMA* 2001; **285**: 785–95.

5 World Health Organization (WHO). *Assessment of Fracture Risk and its Application to Screening for Postmenopausal Osteoporosis.* WHO Technical Report Series No. 843. Geneva: WHO, 1994.

6 Poole KES, Compston JE. Osteoporosis and its management. *BMJ* 2006; **333**: 1251–6.

7 Black DM, Palermo L, Grima DT. Developing better economic models of osteoporosis: considerations for the calculation of the relative risk of fracture. *Value Health* 2006; **9**: 54–8.

8 Committee on Safety of Medicines. Further advice on safety of HRT: risk:benefit unfavourable for first-line use in prevention of osteoporosis. CEM/CMO/2003/19, 2003. www.mhra.gov.uk (accessed 18 09 07)

9 National Institute for Health and Clinical Excellence (NICE). Osteoporosis guidelines www.nice.org.uk/guidance and http://guidance.nice.org.uk/topic/musculoskeletal/?node=7194&wordid=142 (accessed 18 09 07)

10 Beral V; Million Women Study Collaborators. Breast cancer and hormone-replacement therapy in the Million Women Study. *Lancet* 2003; **362**: 419–27.

11 Rees M, Purdie DW (eds). *Management of the Menopause: The Handbook*, 4th edn. London: Royal Society of Medicine Press, 2006.

12 Kanis JA, Oden A, Johnell O, Johansson H, De Laet C, Brown J, Burckhardt P, Cooper C, Christiansen C, Cummings S, Eisman JA, Fujiwara S, Gluer C, Goltzman D, Hans D, Krieg MA, La Croix A, McCloskey E, Mellstrom D, Melton LJ 3rd, Pols H, Reeve J, Sanders K, Schott AM, Silman A, Torgerson D, van Staa T, Watts NB, Yoshimura N. The use of clinical risk factors enhances the performance of BMD in the prediction of hip and osteoporotic fractures in men and women. *Osteoporos Int* 2007; **18**: 1033–46.

Gynaecological Cancer

PROBLEM

45 Cervical Cancer

Case History

A 32-year-old nulliparous woman undergoes her first cervical Papanicolaou smear test which shows a high-grade squamous intraepithelial lesion (HGSIL). Colposcopy shows an abnormal transformation zone with acetowhite changes and punctation extending into the cervical canal. Biopsy is reported as HGSIL. A cold knife cone biopsy reveals a high-grade squamous cell carcinoma with a depth of invasion of 6 mm and horizontal spread of 8 mm. There is no lymphovascular space invasion (LVSI).

What is the appropriate pre-treatment evaluation for a cervical cancer?

What is the best treatment for a patient with a stage IB1 or early stage IIA cervical cancer?

When is fertility preservation an option in cervical cancer?

What are the indications for adjuvant radiotherapy and when should chemotherapy be added?

Background

Cervical cancer is worldwide the second most common malignancy in women. Introduction of organized screening programmes in industrialized countries has resulted in a noticeable stage shift from more advanced to earlier-stage disease. Small invasive cancers have therefore become a more frequently encountered clinical problem and are often diagnosed at a younger age.

The practical approach to cervical cancer treatment involves three steps: (a) establishing a diagnosis; (b) staging; and (c) choosing and implementing treatment.

What is the appropriate pre-treatment evaluation for a cervical cancer?

Invasive cervical cancer might be encountered when performing colposcopy to evaluate cytological abnormalities. Diagnostic cold knife cone biopsy is indicated when a cancer is suspected and the lesion cannot be fully evaluated (e.g. endocervical extension). When confronted with a clinically evident tumour, an office/outpatient biopsy is sufficient.

Every patient should be formally staged. The current International Federation of Gynaecology and Obstetrics (FIGO) staging system of cervical cancer is based on clinical evaluation and determines surgical resectability of the disease (Table 45.1). Therefore, clinical examination under anaesthesia (EUA) should be performed and suspected bladder or rectal involvement excluded by cystoscopy and/or sigmoidoscopy. Further examination includes intravenous urography and X-ray examination of the lungs and skeleton. Critics of FIGO staging note that EUA is incorrect in a high percentage of cases.[1] Furthermore, substantial data can be obtained from computed tomography (CT), magnetic resonance imaging (MRI), positron emission tomography (PET) and surgical staging. MRI has been increasingly used in cervical cancer and is reported to have a high accuracy in the detection of parametrial involvement and is superior to clinical examination.[2] For assessment of lymph node involvement, however, PET scan is the most accurate and CT scan the most cost-effective imaging procedure.

Table 45.1 FIGO staging for cervical carcinoma	
Stage	
IA1	Microscopic tumour. Stromal invasion ≤3 mm in depth and ≤7 mm in horizontal spread
IA2	Microscopic tumour. Stromal invasion >3 mm and ≤5 mm in depth and ≤7 mm in horizontal spread
IB1	Microscopic lesion >IA2 or clinically visible lesion ≤4 cm in greatest dimension
IB2	Clinically visible lesion >4 cm in greatest dimension
IIA	Extension to upper two-thirds of vagina, no parametrial involvement
IIB	Parametrial involvement but not to pelvic sidewall and no involvement of lower third of vagina
IIIA	Extension to lower third of vagina but not to pelvic sidewall
IVA	Invasion into bladder or rectum
IVB	Distant metastasis

What is the best treatment for a patient with a stage IB1 or early stage IIA cervical cancer?

For FIGO stage IA1 without LVSI, cold knife cone biopsy with clear margins is sufficient since the rate of parametrial and pelvic lymph involvement is negligible. For more advanced cervical cancer, radical hysterectomy including pelvic lymph node dissection or including radiation therapy have traditionally been considered the only standard treatment options. Both treatments result in loss of normal fertility. However, 10%–15% of cervical cancers occur in women during reproductive years, and some of these patients may wish to preserve fertility under all circumstances.

When is fertility preservation an option in cervical cancer?

Radical trachelectomy is a relatively new fertility-sparing surgical technique for selected patients with early cervical cancer (Table 45.2). It involves the removal of the upper vaginal cuff, paracervical ligaments and cervix up to the isthmus. The lower uterine segment is then rejoined to the vagina after the insertion of a permanent cerclage at the level of the isthmus. The procedure may be performed either using a vaginal or abdominal approach and is most commonly combined with a pelvic lymph node dissection.[3] The outcome in terms of overall recurrence and survival for patients with cervical cancer of <2 cm in diameter and without LVSI appears to be similar to the outcome achieved with standard radical hysterectomy.[4] Of those women attempting to become pregnant, about 70% are successful on at least one occasion. Cervical stenosis resulting in menstrual disturbances occurs in up to 15% of cases. Pregnancies after radical trachelectomy should be regarded as high risk as they are associated with a risk of prematurity of 20%. Frequent pre-natal visits are therefore recommended in women who have undergone radical trachelectomy.[5] Caesarean section is the usual mode of delivery as a vaginal delivery would necessitate the removal of the buried cerclage and its reinsertion if further pregnancies are planned.

What are the indications for adjuvant radiotherapy and when should chemotherapy be added?

For patients with early cervical cancer, radical hysterectomy and radiation therapy are believed to be equally effective. However, a number of criteria used by clinicians to select patients for one treatment or the other may bias comparisons. Younger women and those who have relatively small tumours (FIGO stage IB1 and early stage IIA) tend to be preferred for primary surgical treatment. But age should not be considered a contraindication for radical surgery, as morbidity in the elderly is similar to that of younger

Table 45.2 Eligibility criteria for fertility preservation by radical vaginal trachelectomy in cervical cancer

- Desire to preserve fertility
- No clinical evidence of impaired fertility
- FIGO stage IA1 with the presence of LVSI, or FIGO stages IA2 and IB1
- Lesion size ≤2.0 cm without LVSI
- No involvement of the upper endocervical canal as determined by colposcopy and/or MRI
- No evidence of pelvic lymph node metastasis

patients. The two main advantages of primary surgery are (a) preservation of ovarian function, and (b) lack of chronic radiation damage to bladder, bowel and vagina, the latter being associated with detrimental effects on sexual function.[6] However, these advantages are eliminated and the associated radiation toxicity is significantly increased if post-operative radiotherapy has to be administered. Consequently, surgery followed by radiotherapy should be avoided when possible. If adverse factors are present (e.g. tumour >4 cm, suspicion of parametrial involvement during EUA, difficult surgical access due to obesity, or involvement of the lower uterine segment on imaging) and there is doubt whether a patient can be sufficiently treated with surgery alone, primary radiotherapy should be given. Classic indications for radiotherapy after radical hysterectomy include positive or close surgical margins, disease extension into the parametria, and lymph node metastasis. In patients without disease beyond the cervix, a combination of large tumour diameter, outer-third cervical stromal invasion and LVSI is associated with a high risk of recurrence and adjuvant radiotherapy may be beneficial.[7]

Several randomized trials have shown an overall survival advantage for cisplatin-based chemotherapy given concurrently with radiotherapy. These studies included women with stage IB2–stage IVA disease with primary radiotherapy, and women with stage I–stage IIA disease found to have poor prognostic factors (e.g. metastatic disease in pelvic lymph nodes, parametrial disease, or positive surgical margins). Significant survival benefit for concurrent chemo-radiation was found, with the risk of death from cervical cancer being decreased by 30%–50%.[8]

Recent Developments

Virtually all cervical cancers are causally related to infections with the human papillomavirus (HPV). Two distinct prophylactic vaccines against the most common HPV types have been developed. One is made by Merck (Gardasil®) and the other is made by GlaxoSmithKline (Cervarix™). Both vaccines induce antibodies to HPV types 16 and 18, which account for about 70% of all cervical cancers worldwide. The Merck vaccine also incorporates protection against HPV types 6 and 11, which are associated with approximately 90% of genital warts. Numerous trials have been published on the efficacy of these vaccines. The American Cancer Society recommends routine HPV vaccination for females aged 11 to 12 years.[9] A reduction of the cervical cancer risk by 70% or more – depending on the number of carcinogenic HPV types eventually included in a future vaccine – becomes a theoretical possibility. However, vaccinating young girls will not have an impact on the incidence of cervical cancer until they reach the median age of cervical cancer diagnosis of 48 years. Meanwhile, the development of a therapeutic vaccine remains a high priority.

Conclusion

This patient is nulliparous and ideally would like to have children. She elects for fertility-sparing surgery and is aware of the the risk of prematurity and the need for a Caesarean section should she fall pregnant.

Further Reading

1 Narayan K. Arguments for a magnetic resonance imaging-assisted FIGO staging system for cervical cancer. *Int J Gynecol Cancer* 2005; **15**: 573–82.

2 Park W, Park YJ, Huh SJ, Kim BG, Bae DS, Lee J, Kim BH, Choi JY, Ahn YC, Lim DH. The usefulness of MRI and PET imaging for the detection of parametrial involvement and lymph node metastasis in patients with cervical cancer. *Jpn J Clin Oncol* 2005; **35**: 260–4.

3 Abu-Rustum NR, Sonoda Y, Black D, Levine DA, Chi DS, Barakat RR. Fertility-sparing radical abdominal trachelectomy for cervical carcinoma: technique and review of the literature. *Gynecol Oncol* 2006; **103**: 807–13.

4 Plante M, Renaud MC, Francois H, Roy M. Vaginal radical trachelectomy: an oncologically safe fertility-preserving surgery. An updated series of 72 cases and review of the literature. *Gynecol Oncol* 2004; **94**: 614–23.

5 Boss EA, van Golde RJ, Beerendonk CC, Massuger LF. Pregnancy after radical trachelectomy: a real option? *Gynecol Oncol* 2005; **99**: S152–6.

6 Frumovitz M, Sun CC, Schover LR, Munsell MF, Jhingran A, Wharton JT, Eifel P, Bevers TB, Levenback CF, Gershenson DM, Bodurka DC. Quality of life and sexual functioning in cervical cancer survivors. *J Clin Oncol* 2005; **23**: 7428–36.

7 Rotman M, Sedlis A, Piedmonte MR, Bundy B, Lentz SS, Muderspach LI, Zaino RJ. A phase III randomized trial of postoperative pelvic irradiation in Stage IB cervical carcinoma with poor prognostic features: follow-up of a gynecologic oncology group study. *Int J Radiat Oncol Biol Phys* 2006; **65**: 169–76.

8 Eifel PJ. Concurrent chemotherapy and radiation therapy as the standard of care for cervical cancer. *Nat Clin Pract Oncol* 2006; **3**: 248–55.

9 Saslow D, Castle PE, Cox JT, Davey DD, Einstein MH, Ferris DG, Goldie SJ, Harper DM, Kinney W, Moscicki AB, Noller KL, Wheeler CM, Ades T, Andrews KS, Doroshenk MK, Kahn KG, Schmidt C, Shafey O, Smith RA, Partridge EE; Gynecologic Cancer Advisory Group, Garcia F. American Cancer Society Guideline for human papillomavirus (HPV) vaccine use to prevent cervical cancer and its precursors. *CA Cancer J Clin* 2007; **57**: 7–28.

46 Endometrial Cancer

Case History

A 34-year-old nulliparous woman presents with six months' history of irregular menstrual bleeding. She has a body mass index of 35 kg/m^2 and was diagnosed with polycystic ovary syndrome (PCOS) a few years ago. A pipelle biopsy is taken which shows a grade I endometrioid adenocarcinoma.

What is the standard treatment for endometrial cancer?

What is the role of laparoscopy in endometrial cancer?

Can fertility be preserved in endometrial cancer?

What is the optimal type of adjuvant radiotherapy and the role of chemotherapy in endometrial cancer?

Can hormone replacement therapy be given after endometrial cancer?

Table 46.1 FIGO staging for endometrial carcinoma	
Stage	
I	Tumour confined to the corpus
IA	Tumour limited to the endometrium
IB	Tumour invades up to or less than one-half of myometrium
IC	Tumour invades more than one-half of myometrium
II	Tumour involving the cervix
IIA	Endocervical gland involvement only
IIB	Cervical stroma invasion
III	Local and/or regional spread
IIIA	Tumour involves serosa and/or adnexa and/or cancer cells in ascites or washings
IIIB	Vaginal involvement
IIIC	Metastasis to pelvic and/or para-aortic lymph nodes
IV	Involvement of bladder mucosa and/or bowel mucosa and/or distant metastasis
IVA	Tumour involves bladder mucosa and/or bowel mucosa
IVB	Distant metastasis (including intra-abdominal and/or inguinal lymph nodes)

Background

What is the standard treatment for endometrial cancer?

Endometrial cancer is the most common gynaecological cancer in the industrialized world. Standard treatment for early endometrial cancer (International Federation of Gynaecology and Obstetrics [FIGO] stage I; Table 46.1) is surgery consisting of a total abdominal hysterectomy and bilateral salpingo-oophorectomy (Figure 46.1). Peritoneal washings should also be collected and the peritoneal surfaces carefully examined for the presence of tumour implants. Furthermore, pelvic lymph node dissection is advocated by many for diagnostic, therapeutic and prognostic purposes. It facilitates targeted therapy to maximize survival and to minimize the effects of undertreatment and potential morbidity associated with overtreatment (e.g. radiation toxicity). The use of lymphadenectomy – selective node sampling versus formal lymphadenectomy, and pelvic versus pelvic plus para-aortic lymphadenectomy – remains controversial. The American College of Obstetricians and Gynecologists (ACOG) advocates full pelvic and para-aortic lymph node dissection.[1] The incidence and severity of complications associated with extensive surgical staging is low and is most frequently related to the effects of existing medical

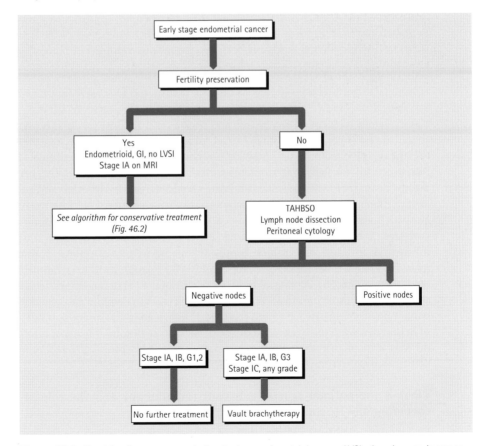

Figure 46.1 Algorithm for management of early stage endometrial cancer. LVSI = lymphovascular space involvement; TAHBSO = total abdominal hysterectomy and bilateral salpingo-oophorectomy.

comorbidities (i.e. obesity, diabetes). The average hospital stay for full staging is similar to that for standard hysterectomy.

What is the role of laparoscopy in endometrial cancer?

There has been a recent trend towards laparoscopic management of early endometrial cancer.[2] Techniques include total laparoscopic hysterectomy and laparoscopic-assisted vaginal hysterectomy. The reputed benefits of laparoscopic surgery are reduced morbidity and shorter recovery time and hospital stay. Laparoscopic-assisted vaginal hysterectomy usually involves laparoscopic securing of the ovarian pedicles and reflection of the bladder and may or may not include laparoscopic division of the uterine vessels before completing the rest of the procedure through the vagina. In contrast, total laparoscopic hysterectomy involves performing the entire operation laparoscopically. A specially designed tube, such as the McCartney tube, is inserted into the vagina to stabilize it, allowing easier dissection of the bladder and exposure of the cervico-vaginal junction. The tube also helps to identify a safe point for division of the uterine vessels and permits maintenance of the pneumoperitoneum once the vagina is opened.[3] Prerequisite for the laparoscopic approach is that staging and extent of surgery is not compromised due to technical issues. The Laparoscopic Surgery or Standard Surgery in Treating Patients With Endometrial Cancer or Cancer of the Uterus (LAP2) trial and the Laparoscopic Approach to Cancer of the Endometrium (LACE) study are currently examining the equivalence of the laparoscopic hysterectomy and the standard open surgical approach in endometrial cancer.[4]

Can fertility be preserved in endometrial cancer?

Hormonal therapy with progestogens can be an alternative to surgery to preserve fertility in selected patients (Figure 46.2). Factors that affect the decision are age, obstetric history, family history and any history and reason for infertility. Optimal cancer therapy should always supersede fertility preservation as the primary objective, and the extent of the disease is the major determinant as to whether fertility-sparing treatment should be recommended. Furthermore, women have to be aware that data are limited, being based on small case series. The optimal candidate should have an early lesion and good prognostic criteria – a stage IA, grade I endometrioid adenocarcinoma without lymphovascular space invasion (LVSI). The histological diagnosis has to be made by hysteroscopy and curettage. Magnetic resonance imaging (MRI) is recommended to assess the depth of myometrial invasion and exclude lymphadenopathy or a synchronous ovarian malignancy. For patients who are eligible for conservative management, a six-month trial with medroxyprogesterone acetate (MPA) (400 mg/day) is undertaken with endometrial curettage every three months. About 70% complete remission and subsequently a pregnancy rate of about 70% have been reported.[5,6] When an initial response is not achieved, or in case of disease recurrence, extension of the disease beyond the uterus is rare. Due to the high incidence of up to 40% of recurrent endometrial disease, it is recommended to perform a hysterectomy once childbearing has been completed.

What is the optimal type of adjuvant radiotherapy and the role of chemotherapy in endometrial cancer?

Radiation is usually given in the adjuvant setting as external beam radiotherapy or vault brachytherapy. With increasing emphasis on complete surgical staging including lymph node dissection, a significant number of patients are found to have tumours with very

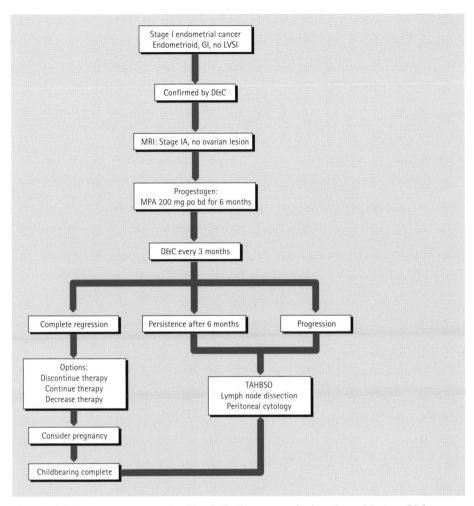

Figure 46.2 Suggested treatment algorithm for fertility preservation in endometrial cancer. D&C = dilatation and curettage; LVSI = lymphovascular space involvement; MPA = medroxyprogesterone acetate; TAHBSO = total abdominal hysterectomy and bilateral salpingo-oophorectomy.

good prognosis (stage IA or IB, grade I or 2 tumours) that do not warrant radiotherapy. The use of adjuvant radiation therapy in more advanced disease limited to the uterus is controversial. In those cases, adjuvant radiotherapy has been shown to significantly reduce the incidence of both pelvic and vaginal recurrence. Nevertheless, evidence to support survival benefit from adjuvant radiotherapy in those cases is poor, as deaths generally result from disease recurrence outside the radiation field. Therefore, many practitioners have abandoned external beam radiotherapy in patients with negative nodes and have replaced it with vault brachytherapy for selected patients with increased risk of vault recurrence. Patients with positive lymph nodes and other extrauterine disease, however, are candidates for external beam radiotherapy. What remains unclear is what represents optimal radiation therapy, and many patients receive a highly individualized approach due to the widely varying manifestations of extrauterine spread.

Cytotoxic chemotherapy has no proven role in the management of early stage endometrial cancer but is used in patients with primary advanced or recurrent endometrial cancer. For those cases, many agents have been studied but only a few have demonstrated significant single-agent activity. The most active single agents appear to be doxorubicin, cisplatin and paclitaxel with response rates of 20%–40%. The combination of doxorubicin and cisplatin produces response rates of about 60%.[7]

Can hormone replacement therapy be given after endometrial cancer?

Hormone replacement therapy (HRT) after endometrial cancer is a controversial topic.[8] Only a few studies have investigated the use of HRT in women with a history of endometrial cancer. They have failed to demonstrate any increase in recurrence or death rate among HRT users and thus its use in endometrial cancer survivors does not seem to be contraindicated.[9] However, the studies are limited by small sample size, retrospective design, selection bias, variation in hormone preparations and disease severity. Therefore, although the available data are encouraging, the question of whether HRT should be given after endometrial cancer remains unanswered. ACOG has stated that there is insufficient evidence to support specific recommendations regarding the use of HRT in women with a history of endometrial cancer. They have commented that, although the indications for use of HRT in this population are similar to those for other women, patients should be selected on the basis of prognostic indicators such as depth of invasion, grading and cell type and the risk the patient is willing to take.[10] In conclusion, the patient's symptoms and quality of life have to be balanced against the potential benefits and adverse effects of HRT, and an individualized patient-based approach must be taken. If a woman elects to try alternative and complementary therapies, she should be advised about the lack of evidence of safety with regard to recurrence.

Recent Developments

1   There has been a recent trend towards laparoscopic management of early endometrial cancer.[2] Techniques include total laparoscopic hysterectomy and laparoscopic-assisted vaginal hysterectomy. The reputed benefits of laparoscopic surgery are reduced morbidity and shorter recovery time and hospital stay. Laparoscopic-assisted vaginal hysterectomy usually involves laparoscopic securing of the ovarian pedicles and reflection of the bladder and may or may not include laparoscopic division of the uterine vessels before completing the rest of the procedure through the vagina. In contrast, total laparoscopic hysterectomy involves performing the entire operation laparoscopically. A specially designed tube, such as the McCartney tube, is inserted into the vagina to stabilize it, allowing easier dissection of the bladder and exposure of the cervico-vaginal junction. The tube also helps to identify a safe point for division of the uterine vessels and permits maintenance of the pneumoperitoneum once the vagina is opened.[3] A prerequisite for the laparoscopic approach is that staging and extent of surgery is not compromised due to technical issues. The Laparoscopic Surgery or Standard Surgery in Treating Patients With Endometrial Cancer or Cancer of the Uterus (LAP2) trial and the Laparoscopic Approach to Cancer of the Endometrium (LACE) study are currently examining the equivalence of the

laparoscopic hysterectomy and the standard open surgical approaches in endometrial cancer.[4]

2   An even more innovative approach to endometrial cancer is the use of robotics. The daVinci Surgical System (Intuitive Surgical Inc., Sunnyvale, CA, USA) was approved by the Food and Drug Administration (FDA) for hysterectomies and latest results show that robotic surgery improves upon laparoscopic treatment of endometrial cancer.[11]

Conclusion

This patient might be a candidate for fertility preservation with progestogens if the hysteroscopy and curettage confirms grade I disease and the MRI shows disease limited to the endometrium. However, she must be made aware that data regarding response rate and outcome are scant. If this patient has to undergo a total abdominal hysterectomy, bilateral salpingo-oophorectomy and pelvic lymph node dissection she could be offered laparoscopic surgery. After surgery she will undergo premature menopause and HRT will be advised until the average of the natural menopause.

Further Reading

1   Hernandez E; American College of Obstetricians and Gynecologists. ACOG Practice Bulletin number 65: management of endometrial cancer. *Obstet Gynecol* 2005; **107**: 952.

2   Schlaerth AC, Abu-Rustum NR. Role of minimally invasive surgery in gynecologic cancers. *Oncologist* 2006; **11**: 895–901.

3   McCartney AJ, Obermair A. Total laparoscopic hysterectomy with a transvaginal tube. *J Am Assoc Gynecol Laparosc* 2004; **11**: 79–82.

4   United States National Institutes of Health. National Library of Medicine. www.clinicaltrials.gov (accessed 20 09 07)

5   Farthing A. Conserving fertility in the management of gynaecological cancers. *BJOG* 2006; **113**: 129–34.

6   Niwa K, Tagami K, Lian Z, Onogi K, Mori H, Tamaya T. Outcome of fertility-preserving treatment in young women with endometrial carcinomas. *BJOG* 2005; **112**: 317–20.

7   Carey MS, Gawlik C, Fung-Kee-Fung M, Chambers A, Oliver T. Systematic review of systemic therapy for advanced or recurrent endometrial cancer. *Gynecol Oncol* 2006; **101**: 158–67.

8   McDonnell BA, Twiggs LB. Hormone replacement therapy in endometrial cancer survivors: new perspectives after the heart and estrogen progestin replacement study and the women's health initiative. *J Low Genit Tract Dis* 2006; **10**: 92–101.

9   Barakat RR, Bundy BN, Spirtos NM, Bell J, Mannel RS. Randomized double-blind trial of estrogen replacement therapy versus placebo in stage I or II endometrial cancer: a Gynecologic Oncology Group Study. *J Clin Oncol* 2006; **24**: 587–92.

10 Committee on Gynecologic Practice. ACOG committee opinion. Hormone replacement therapy in women treated for endometrial cancer. Number 234, May 2000 (replaces number 126, August 1993). *Int J Gynaecol Obstet* 2001; **73**: 283–4.

11 Boggess J.F. Robotic surgery in gynecologic oncology: evolution of a new surgical paradigm. *J Robotic Surg* 2007; **1**: 31–7.

47 Ovarian Cancer

Case History

A 43-year-old woman presents with pelvic pain, urinary frequency and bloating for two months. On pelvic examination she has a normal-sized uterus, deviated posteriorly by a prominent smooth anterior mass. There is no nodularity in the cul-de-sac. A vaginal ultrasound scan reveals a 10 cm mixed solid and cystic right adnexal mass. There is some free fluid. A computed tomography (CT) scan of the abdomen and pelvis confirms the findings. There are no peritoneal implants, omental changes or lymphadenopathy. The serum CA125 level is 150 U/ml. The patient does not have any family history of cancer.

How do you assess the risk of malignancy of an ovarian mass?

What is the optimal surgical management for an apparent early stage ovarian cancer?

What is the role of laparoscopic staging in ovarian cancer?

When can fertility be preserved in ovarian cancer?

What is the optimal management for patients with inadvertent discovery of ovarian cancer ?

Background

How do you assess the risk of malignancy of an ovarian mass?

When a woman presents with a pelvic mass it is important (a) to distinguish between gynaecological and non-gynaecological pathology, and (b) to determine whether the mass is benign or malignant. The best way to detect an early ovarian cancer is to have a high index of suspicion of the diagnosis in a symptomatic woman. A series of warning signs on clinical assessment, blood tests (serum CA125 level) and imaging points to the diagnosis of a malignancy. Most women with ovarian cancer will report symptoms; however, most of them are usually not gynaecological in nature (Table 47.1). It is very important to take a careful clinical history keeping in mind that the risk of ovarian cancer is related to older age and a family history (positive for breast or ovarian cancer). Physical examination is another cornerstone in the assessment and must not be neglected in favour of blood studies or radiology. If on clinical examination there is the suspicion of a mass, a pelvic ultrasound scan should be able to confirm the diagnosis. Ultrasound features that suggest a malignancy include septations, papillary projections, solid areas and

Table 47.1 Ovarian cancer symptoms

- Increased abdominal girth
- Abdominal bloating
- Indigestion, lack of appetite
- Change in bowel habits, including constipation
- Urinary frequency
- Fatigue
- Abdominal and/or pelvic pain

ascites. The presence of ascites has a positive predictive value of 95% for a malignancy. However, less than 20% of early stage ovarian cancers have ascites present. An elevated serum CA125 level can confirm the suspicion of ovarian cancer in a post-menopausal woman. A normal level, however, cannot be taken as a guarantee against malignancy, since about 25% of ovarian carcinomas are marker negative. Furthermore, especially in pre-menopausal women, a large range of gynaecological pathological conditions are known to elevate serum CA125 levels including endometriosis, pelvic inflammatory disease and fibroids.

Efforts to standardize the information obtained from a patient with a pelvic mass have resulted in the development of the 'Risk of Malignancy Index' scoring system which can be used as a method of triage for women with pelvic masses (Table 47.2).[1] The algorithm includes assessment of the woman's menopausal status, the ultrasonographic features and the serum CA125 level. An index score cut-off value of 200 used to discriminate benign from malignant ovarian masses has a sensitivity of 80%, specificity of 92% and positive predictive value of 83%.[2]

Table 47.2 Risk of Malignancy Index

Criteria	Scoring system	Score
Menopausal status		
Pre-menopausal	1	
Post-menopausal	3	A (1 or 3)
Ultrasonographic features		
Multiloculated		
Solid areas	No features = 0	
Bilaterality	1 feature = 1	B (0,1 or 3)
Ascites	>1 feature = 3	
Metastasis		
Serum CA125 level	Absolute levels	C
Risk of Malignancy Index		A × B × C

What is the optimal surgical management for an apparent early stage ovarian cancer?

A woman with a suspicious adnexal mass requires surgical exploration. The goal is to remove the mass safely without rupture and, if malignancy is confirmed, to provide surgical staging to define the extent of the disease (Table 47.3). As scar size, post-operative recovery and cost-effectiveness influence the decision-making process nowadays, a laparoscopic approach can be a reasonable option if the tumour can be removed safely and without rupture. Once the diagnosis of ovarian cancer has been made, a midline laparotomy and surgical staging are mandatory. Access to the upper abdomen is imperative and this cannot be achieved by a Pfannenstiel incision.

Table 47.3 FIGO staging for ovarian carcinomas

Stage	
I	Growth limited to the ovaries
IA	Growth limited to one ovary; no ascites containing malignant cells. No tumour on the external surface; capsule intact
IB	Growth limited to both ovaries; no ascites containing malignant cells. No tumour on the external surface; capsules intact
IC	Tumour either stage IA or IB, but with tumour on the surface of one or both ovaries, or with capsule ruptured, or with ascites present containing malignant cells, or with positive peritoneal washings
II	Pelvic extension
IIA	Extension and/or metastases to the uterus and/or tubes
IIB	Extension to other pelvic tissues
IIC	Tumour either stage IIA or IIB, but with tumour on the surface of one or both ovaries, or with capsules ruptured, or with ascites present containing malignant cells, or with positive peritoneal washings
III	Peritoneal implants outside the pelvis and/or positive retroperitoneal or inguinal nodes and/or extension to small bowel and/or involvement of the omentum
IIIA	Microscopic peritoneal seeding of the abdominal peritoneal surfaces
IIIB	Implants on the abdominal peritoneal surfaces, none exceeding 2 cm in diameter
IIIC	Abdominal implants >2 cm in diameter and/or positive retroperitoneal or inguinal nodes
IV	Distant metastasis. Pleural effusion with positive cytology

What is the role of laparoscopic staging in ovarian cancer?

Laparoscopy, although recently described as a feasible approach for early ovarian cancer staging, is still experimental.[3] Optimal staging for ovarian cancer involves inspection and palpation of all peritoneal surfaces, peritoneal washings, total hysterectomy, bilateral salpingo-oophorectomy, omentectomy, peritoneal biopsies of any suspicious lesions for metastases or blind peritoneal biopsies in the absence of macroscopic disease, and at least an adequate sampling of pelvic and para-aortic lymph nodes. This is laparoscopically not feasible. An optimal surgical staging is achieved in 97% of cases if surgery is performed by an experienced gynaecological oncologist compared with a gynaecologist (53%) or a general surgeon (35%) and is known to be associated with a better survival.[4]

When can fertility be preserved in ovarian cancer?

Pre-menopausal women who wish to retain their fertility may have fertility-preserving surgery/staging (preservation of uterus and contralateral ovary) if they have early stage disease and favourable low-risk pathology (Table 47.4). This approach is appropriate only if an otherwise thorough staging has confirmed no extra-ovarian spread.[5] In cases with fertility-preserving surgery, the patient should undergo three-monthly serum CA125 measurements and the remaining ovary should be monitored with transvaginal ultrasonography every six months. Removing the contralateral ovary should be considered when childbearing has been completed.

Table 47.4 Risk of recurrence in early ovarian cancer	
Risk	**Risk factors**
Low risk	Stage IA or stage IB
	Grade 1 or 2
High risk	All stage I, G3 tumours
	Stage IC (not based on intra-operative cyst rupture)
	Stage IA or IB, Grade 1 or 2 with dense adhesions
	Clear cell carcinomas
	Incompletely staged, apparent early stage tumours

What is the optimal management for patients with inadvertent discovery of ovarian cancer?

There may be circumstances when the diagnosis of ovarian cancer is made unexpectedly at the time of laparotomy. In the case of exploration and an unexpected finding of an ovarian cancer, the so-called 'peek and shriek', a gynaecological oncologist should be consulted intra-operatively. If not available, the diagnosis should be confirmed by appropriate biopsy such as of the omentum and the acute situation dealt with (for example, relief of a bowel obstruction). Otherwise, minimal surgery should be carried out and the patient should be referred to a gynaecological oncology unit (Table 47.5).

Table 47.5 Management of inadvertent diagnosis of ovarian cancer
● Consultation of a gynaecological oncologist intra-operatively
● Confirmation of diagnosis by biopsy
● Management of the acute situation (e.g. bowel obstruction)
● Minimal additional surgery
● Post-operative referral to a gynaecological oncology unit

Recent Developments

The current standard of adjuvant care for advanced epithelial ovarian cancer consists of intravenous administration of platinum- and taxane-based chemotherapy. Despite the improved median overall survival in patients receiving such regimens, relapse still occurs in more than 50% of those with advanced disease and only 10%–30% of such patients have long-term survival.[6] Better therapies alone or in combination with those established cytotoxics are therefore warranted. Angiogenesis, the process by which new blood vessels develop from the endothelium of pre-existing vasculature, is a crucial step in the uncontrolled growth, invasion and metastasis of malignancies like ovarian cancer. Several proangiogenic factors may be potential targets for antiangiogenic therapy in ovarian cancer. One of the best studied angiogenic factors is the vascular endothelial growth factor (VEGF). Bevacizumab (Avastin) is a recombinant monoclonal antibody directed against VEGF. The antibody has shown promising antitumour activity in ovarian cancer as a single agent and in combination with chemotherapy in phase II trials.[7] Two ongoing randomized trials are evaluating the benefit of adding bevacizumab to carboplatin and paclitaxel in the first-line setting: GOG218 and ICON7.[8,9]

Conclusion

The size of the ovarian cyst would make it difficult to retrieve it laparoscopically without risk of rupture. Furthermore, the morphological characteristics of the lesion on ultrasound combined with an elevated CA125 and potential ascites add up to a high risk of malignancy index. The patient therefore undergoes an exploratory laparotomy. She is found to have miliary metastatic peritoneal disease on all peritoneal surfaces including the diaphragm. The frozen section of the ovarian mass reveals a high-grade serous papillary carcinoma of the ovary. She undergoes a full staging operation to which she had consented pre-operatively.

Further Reading

1 Jacobs I, Oram D, Fairbanks J, Turner J, Frost C, Grudzinskas JG. A risk of malignancy index incorporating CA 125, ultrasound and menopausal status for the accurate preoperative diagnosis of ovarian cancer. *Br J Obstet Gynaecol* 1990; **97**: 922–9.

2 Tingulstad S, Hagen B, Skjeldestad FE, Onsrud M, Kiserud T, Halvorsen T, Nustad K. Evaluation of a risk of malignancy index based on serum CA125, ultrasound findings and menopausal status in the pre-operative diagnosis of pelvic masses. *Br J Obstet Gynaecol* 1996; **103**: 826–31.

3 Leblanc E, Sonoda Y, Narducci F, Ferron G, Querleu D. Laparoscopic staging of early ovarian carcinoma. *Curr Opin Obstet Gynecol* 2006; **18**: 407–12.

4 Colombo N, Van Gorp T, Parma G, Amant F, Gatta G, Sessa C, Vergote I. Ovarian cancer. *Crit Rev Oncol Hematol* 2006; **60**: 159–79.

5 Zanetta G, Rota S, Chiari S, Bonazzi C, Bratina G, Torri V, Mangioni C. The accuracy of staging: an important prognostic determinator in stage I ovarian carcinoma. A multivariate analysis. *Ann Oncol* 1998; **9**: 1097–101.

6 Berek JS, Hacker NF (eds). *Practical Gynecologic Oncology*, 4th edn. Sydney: Lippincott Williams & Wilkins, 2005.

7 Rosa DD, Clamp AR, Collinson F, Jayson GC. Antiangiogenic therapy for ovarian cancer. *Curr Opin Oncol* 2007; **19**: 497–505.

8 ICON 7: A Gynaecologic InterGroup Trial. www.ctu.mrc.ac.uk/icon7/ (accessed 25 09 07)

9 ClincalTrials.gov. Carboplatin and paclitaxel with or without bevacizumab in treating patients with stage III or stage IV ovarian epithelial or primary peritoneal cancer. www.clinicaltrials.gov/ct/show/NCT00262847 (accessed 25 09 07)

PROBLEM

48 Vulvar Cancer

Case History

A 72-year-old woman is concerned about a vulvar lesion that has caused itching and pain for about twelve months. On examination, a 15 × 10 mm exophytic inflamed lesion is identified on the right labia majora. There is no palpable inguinal lymphadenopathy.

How do you investigate in a patient with a vulvar lesion suspicious for a malignancy?

What is the surgical management of the primary lesion in early vulvar cancer?

When is an inguinal lymph node dissection indicated in vulvar cancer?

Which patients are believed to be suitable for the sentinel lymph node technique?

What are the indications for post-operative radiotherapy in vulvar cancer?

Background

Vulvar cancer accounts for approximately 3%–5% of all gynaecological malignancies and 1% of all cancers in women, with an incidence rate of 1–2/100000. This incidence is ten times higher for women in their seventies. The most common symptom of vulvar cancer is localized pruritus. Other common symptoms are pain, bleeding, discharge and/or a vulvar mass. On examination the lesions may be fleshy, ulcerated or warty in appearance.

How do you investigate in a patient with a vulvar lesion suspicious for a malignancy?

As part of the clinical assessment the inguinal lymph nodes should be evaluated thoroughly to identify groin node metastasis, and a complete pelvic and rectal examination performed to evaluate the extent of disease. Furthermore, a cervical smear should be taken and a colposcopy of the cervix and vagina should follow because of the common associations with squamous lesions of the lower genital tract. Diagnosis is confirmed by a 4 mm Keys punch biopsy under local anaesthetic. The biopsy should include underlying stroma. It is better not to excise the entire lesion as the definitive excision is more difficult to perform. After the diagnosis of an invasive lesion is made, a computed tomography (CT) scan of the groins and pelvis is often helpful in detecting enlarged lymph nodes, especially in the presence of palpable groin nodes. A chest X-ray excludes pulmonary metastasis (Table 48.1).

What is the surgical management of the primary lesion in early vulvar cancer?

The pattern of dissemination of vulvar carcinomas is mainly lymphogenic to the inguinofemoral lymph nodes. Lymph node status is therefore one of the most significant prognostic variables and is an important factor in the surgico-pathological staging of vulvar cancer (Table 48.2). Treatment of vulvar cancer is separated into two categories:

Table 48.1 Investigations for vulvar cancer

- Punch biopsy of the suspicious lesion including the underlying stroma
- Papanicolaou smear of the cervix
- Colposcopy of the cervix and vagina
- CT scan of the groins and pelvis after confirmation of malignancy
- Chest X-ray after confirmation of malignancy

Table 48.2 International Federation of Gynaecology and Obstetrics (FIGO) staging for carcinoma of the vulva

Stage	
I	Lesions 2 cm or less in size confined to vulva and/or perineum; no nodal metastasis
IA	Lesions 2 cm or less in size confined to the vulva or perineum and with stromal invasion no greater than 1.0 mm; no nodal metastasis
IB	Lesions 2 cm or less in size confined to the vulva or perineum and with stromal invasion greater than 1.0 mm; no nodal metastasis
II	Tumour confined to the vulva and/or perineum more than 2 cm in greatest diameter; no nodal metastasis
III	Tumour of any size with (i) adjacent spread to the lower urethra and/or vagina, or the anus, and/or (ii) unilateral groin node metastasis
IVA	Tumour invades any of the following: upper urethra, bladder mucosa, rectal mucosa, pelvic bone, and/or bilateral regional node metastasis
IVB	Any distant metastasis including pelvic lymph nodes

(a) aimed at removing the primary vulvar tumour, and (b) directed at the treatment of the inguinal lymph nodes. Although surgery is the first choice of treatment there is no standard operation and the approach has to be individualized. The emphasis is on performing the most conservative operation consistent with the cure of the disease.[1] A radical local excision rather than a radical vulvectomy is performed in early stage disease to decrease psychosexual morbidity. For localized lesions this operation is as effective as radical vulvectomy in preventing local recurrence. Surgical removal should achieve free margins of 1 cm and the deep margin should be the inferior fascia of the urogenital diaphragm. In vulvar cancer which arises on the background of extensive vulvar intra-epithelial neoplasia, a radical vulvectomy can be the better approach in an elderly patient who has been suffering from chronic itching and pain for a long time to give symptomatic relief and to exclude other areas of invasion.

When is an inguinal lymph node dissection indicated in vulvar cancer?

As for inguinal lymph node management, patients with T1 tumours and ≤1 mm stromal invasion have less than 1% risk of groin node metastasis and do not require a lymphadenectomy.[2] Patients with T1 tumours with >1 mm invasion and T2 lesions need ipsilateral inguinofemoral lymphadenectomy if the lesion is lateral, and bilateral lymphadenectomy if the lesion is midline (<1 cm from midline) or is involving the anterior labia minora (Figure 48.1). Groin dissection may be safely performed through a triple incision approach to improve primary healing. A proper dissection should involve the removal of all inguinal lymph nodes situated above the fascia lata as well as the femoral lymph node group located medial to the femoral vein.

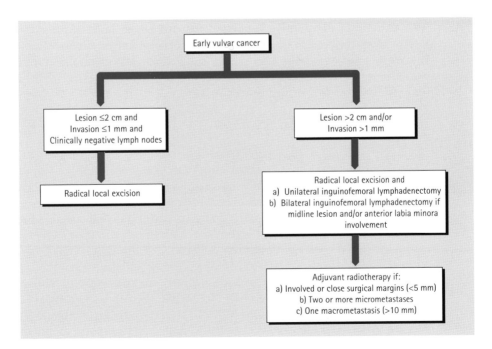

Figure 48.1 Management of early vulvar cancer.

Which patients are believed to be suitable for the sentinel lymph node technique?

One of the major late complications of an inguinal lymph node dissection is chronic leg oedema, which has been reported in up to 69% of patients. This morbidity and the fact that only 20%–30% of patients with clinically unsuspicious inguinofemoral lymph nodes have metastatic lymphatic disease are arguments for the development of minimally invasive methods to be able to omit a complete groin node dissection. The minimally invasive sentinel node procedure is a promising technique for selecting patients for complete lymphadenectomy. The sentinel lymph node is defined as the first draining lymph node, and the pathology of this node is considered to be representative for the lymph nodes it is draining to. Various accuracy studies have shown that the combination of pre-operative peritumoral injection of [99m]technetium-labelled nanocolloid and imaging with the gamma-camera, intra-operative lymphoscintigraphy using a gamma probe, and intra-operative peritumoral injection of blue dye is highly accurate in predicting lymph node metastasis in early vulvar cancer, with a negative predictive value of a negative sentinel lymph node of nearly 100%.[3] Vulvar cancer patients eligible for the sentinel lymph node procedure should be those with (a) histologically proven squamous cell carcinoma of the vulva with depth of invasion >1 mm (>Stage IA), (b) tumours ≤4 cm, (c) no suspicious lymph nodes on inguinal examination, and (d) no enlarged lymph nodes >1.5 cm on a pre-operative magnetic resonance imaging (MRI) or CT scan. At present, the sentinel lymph node procedure is not part of standard care in vulvar cancer as its safety has not yet been proven in a randomized study.[4]

What are the indications for post-operative radiotherapy in vulvar cancer?

After removal of the primary lesion and inguinal lymph node dissection, radiation therapy should be given to help prevent local recurrence and improve survival. It should be given to patients with involved or close surgical margins (<5 mm) and in cases with two or more micrometastases, one macrometastasis (>10 mm) or extracapsular spread in the inguinal lymph nodes (Figure 48.1).[1]

Recent Developments

The common term for vulvar squamous cell carcinoma *in situ* of the vulva is vulvar intraepithelial neoplasia (VIN). VIN has long been classified as VIN1, VIN2, or VIN3 similar to the terminology used for cervical intraepithelial lesions (CIN). However, there is no evidence that VIN and CIN have a similar natural history or that the grading of VIN reflects a biological continuum. It is generally accepted that VIN1 has a very low malignant potential and is not a precursor of VIN2 or VIN3. Futhermore, VIN1 is not a reproducible diagnosis when a lesion is classified by different pathologists and VIN 2 and 3 are not reliably separated.[5] The International Society for the Study of Vulvar Disease (ISSVD) has therefore introduced a new VIN classification in which VIN1 has been eliminated and VIN2 has been combined with VIN3.[6] In the new classification, VIN implies high-grade squamous intraepithelial disease with significant potential for progression to invasive disease requiring excision or destructive therapy (e.g. laser treatment). However, clinicians have to keep in mind that the adoption of the new ISSVD classification is going to take time and it is recommended to communicate with the pathologist if reports of VIN in fact represent high-grade disease.

Conclusion

A punch biopsy of the vulvar lesion under local anaesthetic in the outpatient clinic shows an undifferentiated squamous cell carcinoma. A CT abdo/pelvis and a chest X-ray are performed and both are normal. The patient is consented for a radical right hemivulvectomy and a sentinel lymph node procedure with ^{99m}technetium-labelled nanocolloid. Pre-operative imaging with the gamma-camera after injection of the nanocolloid identifies a single sentinel lymph node in the right groin. A right hemivulvectomy is performed followed by an inguinal incision above the labelled sentinel lymph node which is located with the gamma-counter. The sentinel lymph node is discovered and excised. No other radioactive or pathologically enlarged lymph nodes are identified in the inguinal fossa. The frozen section does not show any tumour involvement of the sentinel lymph node. This is confirmed in the final pathology after the lymph node has been examined by serial sectioning and cytokeratin staining.

Further Reading

1 Berek JS, Hacker NF (eds). *Practical Gynecologic Oncology*, 4th edn. Sydney: Lippincott Williams & Wilkins, 2005.

2 Hacker NF, Van der Velden J. Conservative management of early vulvar cancer. *Cancer* 1993; **71** (4 Suppl): 1673–7.

3 de Hullu JA, Hollema H, Piers DA, Verheijen RH, van Diest PJ, Mourits MJ, Aalders JG, van der Zee AG. Sentinel lymph node procedure is highly accurate in squamous cell carcinoma of the vulva. *J Clin Oncol* 2000; **18**: 2811–16.

4 de Hullu JA, van der Zee AG. Surgery and radiotherapy in vulvar cancer. *Crit Rev Oncol Hematol* 2006; **60**: 38–58.

5 Scurry J, Wilkinson EJ. Review of terminology of precursors of vulvar squamous cell carcinoma. *J Low Genit Tract Dis* 2006; **10**: 161–9.

6 Sideri M, Jones RW, Wilkinson EJ, Preti M, Heller DS, Scurry J, Haefner H, Neill S. Squamous vulvar intraepithelial neoplasia: 2004 modified terminology, ISSVD Vulvar Oncology Subcommittee. *J Reprod Med* 2005; **50**: 807–10.

49 Fallopian Tube Cancer

Case History

A 58-year-old woman is admitted with a two months history of post-menopausal bleeding and abdominal pain. Recto-vaginal examination reveals a right adnexal mass. Computed tomography (CT) of the abdomen shows a mixed solid and cystic right adnexal mass with some ascites but no lymphadenopathy. Serum CA125 level is 950 units/ml. A laparotomy is performed and mass involving the right fallopian tube is identified. The frozen section of the lesion is reported as high-grade fallopian tube carcinoma.

What are the clinical features of a fallopian tube carcinoma?

What is the appropriate surgery for a fallopian tube carcinoma?

How is a fallopian tube carcinoma staged?

What is the current standard of adjuvant care for a fallopian tube carcinoma?

What is the prognosis for patients with a fallopian tube carcinoma?

Background

Fallopian tube carcinomas are the rarest of the gynaecological cancers, accounting for approximately 0.14%–1.8% of female genital malignancies. Epidemiologically, the risk factors for tubal cancer remain obscure, but it is reasonable to presume that hormonal, reproductive and perhaps genetic factors that increase the risk for ovarian carcinoma may also be relevant to fallopian tube cancer. It is part of the *BRCA* mutation phenotype.[1] Therefore, the risk for this malignancy should be considered when prophylactic oophorectomy is performed in high-risk women. The incidence of fallopian tube carcinomas increases with age but peaks at age 60–66 years.

What are the clinical features of a fallopian tube carcinoma?

Patients may present with vaginal bleeding or unexplained vaginal discharge, pelvic pain and a pelvic mass. The presence of pain is significant since cancers of the ovary, endometrium and cervix usually do not cause it. Nevertheless, pre-operative diagnosis of a fallopian tube carcinoma is extremely rare. The classic description of 'hydrops tubae profluens', which is characterized by colicky lower abdominal pain relieved by passing blood-tinged fluid, is rarely spontaneously encountered but is almost pathognomonic. Although serum CA125 level *per se* is not diagnostic for fallopian tube cancers, >80% of patients have elevated pre-treatment values (Table 49.1).[2]

Table 49.1 Typical clinical features of a fallopian tube carcinoma

- Vaginal bleeding or discharge
- Abdominal pain – colicky or dull
- Adnexal/pelvic mass
- Ascites
- Elevated serum CA125

The diagnosis of a fallopian tube carcinoma is usually first made by a pathologist on histopathological examination. Because it is difficult to differentiate between fallopian tube carcinomas and epithelial ovarian carcinomas, at least one of the following criteria should have the diagnosis of fallopian tube carcinoma: (a) grossly, the main tumour is in the tube and arises from the endosalpinx; (b) histologically, the pattern reproduces the epithelium of tubal mucosa and shows a papillary pattern; (c) transition from benign to malignant tubal epithelium should be demonstrated; and (d) the ovaries and endometrium are normal or have a much smaller tumour volume than that of the tube.[3]

What is the appropriate surgery for a fallopian tube carcinoma?

Surgical principles are the same as those used for ovarian cancer. This includes cytological analysis of ascites or pelvic washings, abdominal hysterectomy and bilateral salpingo-oophorectomy, omentectomy, pelvic and para-aortic lymph node dissection and selective peritoneal biopsies. Fallopian tube carcinomas have a strong tendency for lymphatic spread and a full lymph node dissection was reported to be associated with an increased overall survival.[4] In advanced disease, post-operative residual disease >2 cm is an adverse prognostic parameter and therefore full cytoreduction/debulking has to be aimed for.

How is a fallopian tube carcinoma staged?

Staging of fallopian tube carcinomas is based on the surgical findings at laparotomy. The International Federation of Gynecology and Obstetrics (FIGO) epithelial ovarian cancer staging system has been adapted to apply to fallopian tube carcinomas (Table 49.2).

What is the current standard of adjuvant care for a fallopian tube carcinoma?

Due to the propensity for peritoneal spread and the relatively high risk for recurrence despite complete surgical resection, there is a strong rationale for adjuvant treatment for patients with early stage disease. However, very few data are currently available. Patients with stage IA and IB disease might not require adjuvant therapy, as for patients with epithelial ovarian cancer. The current standard of adjuvant care for advanced fallopian tube carcinomas is the same as for epithelial ovarian carcinomas and consists of intravenous administration of platinum-based and taxane-based chemotherapy. The most commonly used standard regimen consists of a combination of carboplatin, at a dose calculated to produce an area under the concentration–time curve of 5–6, with paclitaxel at a dose of 175 mg per square meter of body-surface area over a three-hour period. This

Table 49.2 FIGO staging of fallopian tube carcinoma	
Stage	
I	Tumour confined to the fallopian tubes
IA	Tumour confined to one tube without infiltrating serosal surface
IB	Tumour confined to both tubes without infiltrating serosal surface
IC	Tumour confined to one or both tubes with extension onto serosal surface and/or with positive malignant cells in peritoneal fluid
II	Tumour with pelvic extension
IIA	Extension and/or metastases to uterus and/or ovaries
IIB	Extension to other pelvic organs
IIC	Stage IIA or IIB with positive malignant cells in peritoneal fluid
III	Peritoneal implants outside of the pelvis and/or positive regional lymph nodes
IIIA	Microscopic peritoneal metastases outside the pelvis
IIIB	Macroscopic peritoneal metastases ≤2 cm in greatest dimension
IIIC	Macroscopic peritoneal metastases >2 cm in greatest dimension
IV	Distant metastasis beyond the peritoneal cavity

treatment produces response rates of about 90%, with about 75%–80% of patients having a complete clinical remission. Unfortunately, most women have a relapse of the disease, with only 10%–30% surviving long-term. The addition of maintenance chemotherapy has not improved this discouraging number.

What is the prognosis for patients with a fallopian tube carcinoma?

As described above, prognosis is generally poor. Stage is the most consistent prognostic factor associated with survival. The reported five-year survival rate for patients with stage I disease is 84% versus 36% for stage III disease. The overall five-year survival for patients with fallopian tube carcinomas is 56%. This number is higher than for patients with epithelial ovarian carcinomas and is related to the higher proportion of patients with early stage disease.[5]

Recent Developments

Intraperitoneal chemotherapy (IP) has emerged as an alternative or an addition to intravenous therapy; recent results of the Gynecologic Oncology Group have shown a survival advantage for the use of IP chemotherapy, as compared with a standard intravenous regimen in epithelial ovarian cancer.[6] Although data from intraperitoneal therapy in fallopian tube carcinoma do not exist for large numbers of patients, this type of treatment could possibly be recommended for the management of optimally debulked disease as fallopian tube and ovarian cancers share similar biology.[7] Latest clinical studies on IP chemotherapy (e.g. TRIPOD study) involve patients with both ovarian or tubal cancer.[8]

Conclusion

This patient underwent a full staging laparotomy involving a total abdominal hysterectomy, bilateral salpingo-oophorectomy and omentectomy. The final pathology showed a FIGO stage IIIb fallopian tube carcinoma with several subcentimetre nodules in the omentum. She received six cycles of the carboplatin + paclitaxel combination chemotherapy as adjuvant treatment.

Further Reading

1 Levine DA, Argenta PA, Yee CJ, Marshall DS, Olvera N, Bogomolniy F, Rahaman JA, Robson ME, Offit K, Barakat RR, Soslow RA, Boyd J. Fallopian tube and primary peritoneal carcinomas associated with BRCA mutations. *J Clin Oncol* 2003; **21**: 4222–7.

2 Ajithkumar TV, Minimole AL, John MM, Ashokkumar OS. Primary fallopian tube carcinoma. *Obstet Gynecol Surv* 2005; **60**: 247–52.

3 Hu CY, Taymor ML, Hertig AT. Primary carcinoma of the fallopian tube. *Am J Obstet Gynecol* 1950; **59**: 58–67.

4 Klein M, Rosen AC, Lahousen M, Graf AH, Rainer A. Lymphadenectomy in primary carcinoma of the Fallopian tube. *Cancer Lett* 1999; **147**: 63–6.

5 Heintz AP, Odicino F, Maisonneuve P, Beller U, Benedet JL, Creasman WT, Ngan HY, Sideri M, Pecorelli S. Carcinoma of the Fallopian tube. *J Epidemiol Biostat* 2001; **6**: 89–103.

6 Armstrong DK, Bundy B, Wenzel L, Huang HQ, Baergen R, Lele S, Copeland LJ, Walker JL, Burger RA. Intraperitoneal cisplatin and paclitaxel in ovarian cancer. *N Engl J Med* 2006; **354**: 34–43.

7 Pectasides D, Pectasides E, Economopoulos T. Fallopian tube carcinoma: a review. *Oncologist* 2006; **11**: 902–12.

8 TRIPOD Study. www.anzgog.org.au/trialdetails.aspx?trialno=5 (accessed 29 09 07)

50 Prophylactic Salpingo-oophorectomy

Case History

A 36-year-old woman has a history of familial cancer including her mother and a sister, both with ovarian cancer diagnosed at age 57 and 46 years, respectively, and an aunt on her mother's side with breast cancer diagnosed at age 37 years. She asks you for advice with regard to prophylactic surgery to decrease her risk of developing ovarian cancer.

Who should be offered a prophylactic salpingo-oophorectomy?

What is the optimal timing for a prophylactic salpingo-oophorectomy?

How should a prophylactic salpingo-oophorectomy be performed?

How do you manage women following risk-reducing salpingo-oophorectomy?

Background

Who should be offered a prophylactic salpingo-oophorectomy?

Bilateral salpingo-oophorectomy is an option for reducing the risk of ovarian cancer in women with hereditary predisposition for this malignancy. Familial or inherited syndromes account for approximately 10% of cases of ovarian cancer. Familial cancer syndromes associated with ovarian cancer are the (a) breast–ovarian cancer syndrome, and (b) hereditary non-polyposis colorectal cancer syndrome (HNPCC).

The most common hereditary syndrome is the breast–ovarian cancer syndrome which is caused by germline mutations of the tumour suppressor genes *BRCA1* and *BRCA2*. *BRCA1* mutation carriers have an up to 60% lifetime risk of ovarian cancer and an up to 80% lifetime risk of breast cancer. The lifetime risk for *BRCA2* mutation carriers to develop ovarian cancer is up to 40%, the risk for breast cancer up to 80%. In addition, *BRCA* mutations predispose for the development of fallopian tube and primary peritoneal carcinomas and might be associated with serous papillary carcinomas of the endometrium.

Women with documented *BRCA1* or *BRCA2* mutations who undergo risk-reducing salpingo-oophorectomy have a 80%–96% reduction in the risk of ovarian and fallopian tube cancer.[1,2] Furthermore, if the operation is performed before the menopause, it is associated with a 50%–68% reduction in the risk of developing breast cancer. Therefore, there is clear evidence to support offering risk-reducing salpingo-oophorectomy to women with known mutations in *BRCA1* or *BRCA2*.[3]

What is the optimal timing for a prophylactic salpingo–oophorectomy?

For women with *BRCA1* mutations, the risk of ovarian cancer begins to rise in the late 30s and early 40s; for women with *BRCA2* mutations, approximately ten years later. For *BRCA1* mutation carriers, risk-reducing salpingo-oophorectomy should therefore be offered after completion of childbearing at age 35 to 40 years. Although the risk of ovarian cancer for women with *BRCA2* mutation is only up to 3% by age 50 years, the risk of breast cancer at this age may be as high as 34%. To postpone risk-reducing salpingo-oophorectomy until menopause may therefore cause a substantial loss of protection against breast cancer which prophylactic surgery provides.[3] Therefore a prophylactic salpingo-oophorectomy for a *BRCA2* mutation carrier is advisable at age 40 to 45 years.

How should a prophylactic salpingo–oophorectomy be performed?

The minimum operation required for risk reduction in *BRCA* mutation carriers is a bilateral salpingo-oophorectomy. This can be performed by laparotomy or laparoscopy; however, the latter is usually preferable due to lesser morbidity. Peritoneal lavage and cytologic examination might also be advisable as occult ovarian and tubal cancers have been detected in 2%–10% of *BRCA1* mutation carriers undergoing risk-reducing surgery. It is important that the entire ovaries and fallopian tubes are serially sectioned during the pathologic examination so that microscopic lesions are not missed.

It is not clear if a hysterectomy should be part of surgical risk reduction in *BRCA* mutation carriers. The fallopian tube is at risk of malignant transformation in the breast–ovarian cancer syndrome and a substantial part of the intramural fallopian tube remains *in situ* after a bilateral salpingo-oophorectomy, presumably with a residual risk of cancer in this remnant.[4] Futhermore, it has been suggested that *BRCA* mutation is associated with an increased risk for a serous papillary carcinoma of the endometrium[5] and mutation carriers might therefore benefit from a hysterectomy. Finally, a hysterectomy would mean that oestrogen-alone hormone replacement therapy (HRT) can be used, which has a reduced risk of breast cancer compared to combined therapy.[6] Also there would be no risk of endometrial malignancy should the woman require tamoxifen treatment for breast cancer. However, a hysterectomy is associated with increased morbidity, mortality and expense. Thus, as there is no clear clinical evidence for the benefit of hysterectomy in *BRCA* mutation carriers, decisions have to be individualized.

HNPCC is a cancer susceptibility syndrome caused by a germline mutation in one of the DNA-mismatch repair genes. It is associated with the development of multiple types of cancer, including cancer of the ovary, endometrium and large bowel. The lifetime risk of ovarian cancer for a woman with HNPCC is about 10%; the risk for endometrial cancer 40% to 60%.

There is clear evidence of efficacy for prophylactic surgery in women with HNPCC.[7] In view of the high risk for endometrial cancer, women with a predisposition to this syndrome would benefit most from a total abdominal hysterectomy and bilateral salpingo-oophorectomy (TAHBSO). Given the average age at diagnosis of gynaecological cancers, it is reasonable to offer prophylactic surgery to women from age 35 years[8] or five years before the age of the youngest affected family member.

For unaffected women with a significant family history of ovarian cancer without known germline mutation in the family, less information is available regarding the risks and benefits of a prophylactic salpingo-oophorectomy. These women should be referred for genetic counselling and should be managed by a multidisciplinary team of gynaeco-logical oncologists and geneticists experienced in the care of women with familial cancer risk.[3] The potential harms, benefits and limitations of genetic testing need to be considered.

In general, a woman with two first- or second-degree relatives on the same side of the family diagnosed with epithelial ovarian cancer, especially if additional cases of breast cancer are diagnosed before the age of 40 years, has a potentially high lifetime risk of developing ovarian cancer which is between 1 in 30 and 1 in 3. Individual risk may be higher or lower if genetic results are known.[9]

How do you manage women following risk-reducing salpingo-oophorectomy?

A premature surgical menopause is associated with menopausal symptoms and increased risk of cardiovascular disease and osteoporotic fracture. Mortality is significantly higher in women who undergo prophylactic bilateral oophorectomy before the age of 45 years and do not take oestrogen (see Case 12: Premature Menopause). However, the evidence with regard to management of women following risk-reducing salpingo-oophorectomy is lim-ited. HRT has been recommended until the age of 50 years in women with *BRCA1/2* mutations undergoing prophylactic oophorectomy.[10] Also, women with a premature sur-gical menopause may require different doses of oestrogen to control their symptoms com-pared to women with a natural menopause.[11] Data from large studies about the effect of HRT on the decrease in the breast cancer risk reduction after prophylactic salpingo-oophorectomy are awaited. The patient must be counselled about this before surgery.

With regard to the cancer risk after prophylactic salpingo-oophorectomy, *BRCA* mutation carriers continue to have an increased risk of developing breast cancer and require regular breast screening. It is unclear, however, if those women benefit from con-tinued screening for other malignancies. It is estimated that the residual lifetime risk for a peritoneal cancer after salpingo-oophorectomy is about 5%. Serum CA125 determin-ations might therefore have a role for follow-up but the efficacy of this approach is unknown.[3] Women who have had a prophylactic TAHBSO for HNPCC require regular surveillance to exclude non-gynaecological HNPCC-associated malignancies. They might also benefit from further prophylactic surgery such as colectomy.

Recent Developments

There is an ongoing controversy surrounding the pros and cons of a salpingo-oophorec-tomy for prophylactic reasons in women with average risk for ovarian cancer during surgery for benign disease. Some authors argue that ovarian conservation until the age of 65 benefits long-term survival as it decreases the risk from cardiovascular events and hip fractures due to continuous hormone production and this overweighs the decreased risk of mortality from ovarian cancer.[12] However, it is difficult to compare mortality from cardiovascular events and hip fractures with cancer mortality. Cardiovascular disease can be prevented by cholesterol-lowering medication (e.g. statins) and hip fractures can be avoided by treatment of osteoporosis (e.g. exercise, bisphosphonates) or prophylactic measures (e.g. calcium and vitamin D). The mortality of both health problems could be reduced significantly by awareness, change of lifestyle and compliance with treatment. In contrast, there is no prevention for ovarian cancer but oophorectomy. Therefore, from the gynaecological oncological perspective, where benign gynaecological pathology requires surgery in post-menopausal women, a salpingo-oophorectomy should be the preferred option.

Conclusion

 This patient would benefit from genetic counselling. She has a high lifetime risk of developing ovarian cancer which is in between 1 in 30 and 1 in 3 or even higher if a germline mutation is identified in the family. Her family history is consistent with breast–ovarian cancer syndrome. Unless a cancer susceptibility syndrome is identified and she is found not to be a mutation carrier she should have a bilateral salpingo-oophrectomy at age 40.

Further Reading

1 Rebbeck TR, Lynch HT, Neuhausen SL, Narod SA, Van't Veer L, Garber JE, Evans G, Isaacs C, Daly MB, Matloff E, Olopade OI, Weber BL. Prophylactic oophorectomy in carriers of *BRCA1* or *BRCA2* mutations. *N Engl J Med* 2002; **346**: 1616–22.

2 Finch A, Beiner M, Lubinski J, Lynch HT, Moller P, Rosen B, Murphy J, Ghadirian P, Friedman E, Foulkes WD, Kim-Sing C, Wagner T, Tung N, Couch F, Stoppa-Lyonnet D, Ainsworth P, Daly M, Pasini B, Gershoni-Baruch R, Eng C, Olopade OI, McLennan J, Karlan B, Weitzel J, Sun P, Narod SA. Salpingo-oophorectomy and the risk of ovarian, fallopian tube, and peritoneal cancers in women with a *BRCA1* or *BRCA2* mutation. *JAMA* 2006; **296**: 185–92.

3 Society of Gynecologic Oncologists Clinical Practice Committee Statement on Prophylactic Salpingo-oophorectomy. *Gynecol Oncol* 2005; **98**: 179–81.

4 Gerritzen LH, Grefte JM, Hoogerbrugge N, Bulten J, Massuger LF, de Hullu JA. A substantial part of the fallopian tube is left after standard prophylactic bilateral salpingo-oophorectomy. *Int J Gynecol Cancer* 2006; **16**: 1940–4.

5 Lavie O, Hornreich G, Ben-Arie A, Rennert G, Cohen Y, Keidar R, Sagi S, Lahad EL, Auslander R, Beller U. BRCA germline mutations in Jewish women with uterine serous papillary carcinoma. *Gynecol Oncol* 2004; **92**: 521–4.

6 Anderson GL, Limacher M, Assaf AR, Bassford T, Beresford SA, Black H, Bonds D, Brunner R, Brzyski R, Caan B, Chlebowski R, Curb D, Gass M, Hays J, Heiss G, Hendrix S, Howard BV, Hsia J, Hubbell A, Jackson R, Johnson KC, Judd H, Kotchen JM, Kuller L, LaCroix AZ, Lane D, Langer RD, Lasser N, Lewis CE, Manson J, Margolis K, Ockene J, O'Sullivan MJ, Phillips L, Prentice RL, Ritenbaugh C, Robbins J, Rossouw JE, Sarto G, Stefanick ML, Van Horn L, Wactawski-Wende J, Wallace R, Wassertheil-Smoller S; Women's Health Initiative Steering Committee. Effects of conjugated equine estrogen in postmenopausal women with hysterectomy: the Women's Health Initiative randomized controlled trial. *JAMA* 2004; **291**: 1701–12.

7 Schmeler KM, Lynch HT, Chen LM, Munsell MF, Soliman PT, Clark MB, Daniels MS, White KG, Boyd-Rogers SG, Conrad PG, Yang KY, Rubin MM, Sun CC, Slomovitz BM, Gershenson DM, Lu KH. Prophylactic surgery to reduce the risk of gynecologic cancers in the Lynch syndrome. *N Engl J Med* 2006; **354**: 261–9.

8 Lindor NM, Petersen GM, Hadley DW, Kinney AY, Miesfeldt S, Lu KH, Lynch P, Burke W, Press N. Recommendations for the care of individuals with an inherited predisposition to Lynch syndrome: a systematic review. *JAMA* 2006; **296**: 1507–17.

9 National Breast Cancer Centre (NBCC), Australia. *Advice about familial aspects of breast cancer and ovarian cancer: a guide for health professionals.* Camperdown, NSW: NBCC, 2006. www.nbcc.org.au/bestpractice/ (accessed 02 10 07)

10 Armstrong K, Schwartz JS, Randall T, Rubin SC, Weber B. Hormone replacement therapy and life expectancy after prophylactic oophorectomy in women with *BRCA1/2* mutations: a decision analysis. *J Clin Oncol* 2004; **22**: 1045–54.

11 Madalinska JB, van Beurden M, Bleiker EM, Valdimarsdottir HB, Hollenstein J, Massuger LF, Gaarenstroom KN, Mourits MJ, Verheijen RH, van Dorst EB, van der Putten H, van der Velden K, Boonstra H, Aaronson NK. The impact of hormone replacement therapy on menopausal symptoms in younger high-risk women after prophylactic salpingo-oophorectomy. *J Clin Oncol* 2006; **24**: 3576–82.

12 Parker WH, Broder MS, Liu Z, Shoupe D, Farquhar C, Berek JS. Ovarian conservation at the time of hysterectomy for benign disease. *Obstet Gynecol* 2005; **106**: 219–26.

Index

Problem Solving in Women's Health